SOLO
MUMS
MATTER

SOLO MUMS MATTER
WORDS FROM THE HEART

"Normalizing taking care of yourself, just as much as you take care of others."—*Latoya Hamm Wilson*

"And some days life is just hard. And some days are just rough. And some days you just gotta cry before you move forward. And all that is okay."—*Unknown*

"In the symphony of single motherhood, every heartbeat is a testament to love's infinite strength."—*Zoe Gray*

"As a single mum you'll discover inner strengths and capabilities you never knew you had."—*Emma-Louise Smith*

"But being a perfect parent is impossible and attempting to be one can lead to exhaustion. Our research suggests that whatever allows parents to recharge their batteries, to avoid exhaustion, is good for children."—*Moira Mikolajczak*

"Don't feel guilty about being a single mother. Patience is super important as a single mother. You do have to be a little more patient because all the responsibility is on you…ask for help!"—*Nia Long*

"Stay close to the small and free things that comfort your soul."—*Lalah Delia*

"*Solo Mums Matter* is an invaluable resource for single mothers, offering practical advice, heartfelt encouragement, and empowering strategies. Jo-Anne's wisdom and insight, drawn from her own experiences, inspires readers to take charge of their well-being, and reminds us that we deserve to thrive – not just survive!

Having navigated life as a single mum for over a decade and whilst holding down a demanding job, I know first-hand how easy it is to put your own needs last. This book beautifully reinforces the importance of self-care and personal growth; helping preserve your personal identity and create a fulfilling life for both you and your children.

Solo Mums Matter is more than just a guide, it's a lifeline for those seeking balance amidst the challenges of single motherhood. Highly Recommend."

—*Claire McIlroy. Solo Mum, Human Resources Manager.*

SOLO MUMS MATTER

From Compassion Fatigue to
Restoration and Flourishing

JO-ANNE HENDERSON

LD

Published 2025
by LIFE DANCE

ISBN 978-0-473-74771-8 (International Edition)

© Copyright Jo-Anne Henderson 2025

COPYPRESS

Designed by CopyPress, Nelson, New Zealand.

{REAL**NZBOOKS**}

Distributed in New Zealand by Real NZ Books, Nelson, New Zealand.

www.copypress.co.nz

Being a mum to my daughter is the most treasured and important role in my life. I am very blessed in being her mum and to have her as my daughter. As a woman I am many things and must look after myself well so that I fulfil this treasured role; along with the other roles that I want to fulfil in my life. This means treasuring myself.

Jo-Anne Henderson

"I would say to any single parent currently feeling the weight of stereotype or stigmatization that I am prouder of my years as a single mother than any other part of my life."

JK Rowling

I Warmly Dedicate This Book

This is for all the women out there doing it alone raising their children day to day in the best way that they can. We absolutely need to acknowledge the amazing job that we do in the circumstances we are in, with what we have, and must not forget ourselves. Self-compassion is a must.

To my mother who raised me through challenges.

To my sister who also became a solo mum. We shared our challenges and supported each other.

To my friends who were and are a great support to us. They are my New Zealand family – Kim and Chris Charteris-Wright, Nicola and Brian McGrouther, Phillipa Wilson, Rose MacKinnon, Ian and Suzanne Thurlow.

To my two dear friends who prior to passing away gave me a grounding to help me with what was to come. Angela Hourihane and Lynn Campbell.

Michelle Locke, the Founder of Wu Tao – The Dancing Way.

To my Healing Touch mentors and instructors (Healing Touch New Zealand) who were with me along this journey, supporting me through my training and growth through this period. Annis Parker and Deb Carter.

To Pearl, our black Labrador, who was my daughter's dog really. Pearl bed-hopped and snuggled into our tummies to soothe us through the most difficult nights.

Contents

Introduction

Welcome to *Solo Mums Matter: From Compassion Fatigue to Restoration and Flourishing*. Thank you for venturing into reading this book. I am so glad you are here and send a warm, heartfelt hello from one solo mum to another.

My name is Jo-Anne Henderson, and I was born in Yorkshire, UK and moved to New Zealand at the age of 33. Amongst my love of flowers, I am really a dancer at heart. I found that music moved me from an early age and was a staple in my life between the ages of eight and 18 years. This took the form of various dance classes, exams and performances. Playing often equated to bopping through the Radio 1 Top 40 on a Sunday night (that's a lot of dancing) and choreographing routines with two friends to the likes of 'My Camera Never Lies' and 'Land of Make Believe' by Bucks Fizz! Once I left home and went to study, dance sadly fell by the wayside for many years. It's interesting that later in life during a crisis I went back to it, and it was significant in my healing along with a lengthy stint receiving counselling. I now dance pretty much every morning for the love of it and my self-care.

This book is a culmination of the last five years of my 28-year career as an occupational therapist when I developed and ran fatigue management education and support groups in a neuro rehabilitation setting. This latter part of my career coincided with navigating through a spiritual crisis, training in a form of dance movement therapy with foundations in traditional Chinese medicine called The Dancing Way, training to become a Healing Touch practitioner through a divorce and becoming a single mum to my beautiful teenage daughter. When put in a nutshell like that and I read it back, I recognise that it has been quite a journey since my arrival in New Zealand.

I began writing this book before my marriage ended, when I started reading *The Artist's Way* by Julia Cameron – a 12-week course in the form of a book on unblocking the artist inside you. It really is about creating your life. I would wake in the night with inspiration for sections of a book and would write it down straight away so as not to forget. The subjects were related to energy management and self-care. Since then, it had been sitting in the filing cabinet for nine years until the time was right to complete it. It appears that I needed to wait until I went through a divorce and became a solo mum to finish writing it.

The saying 'everything that happens is meant to happen for a reason' has really come to the fore, and in hindsight now gives comfort. The knack is to trust this when you are going through it. I wouldn't have met a gentleman four years down the track who is also a writer and now my partner, if I hadn't gone through tough times.

I want to mention an example of 'everything happens for a reason'. About six months after our initial separation, my daughter Emily asked if we could go back to England for a while. She explained that she wanted to connect with all her grandparents. I thought about how we could do that financially. The money from the sale of the house was held at the solicitors until our divorce was settled. I would need to go through the lawyers to negotiate the release of some funds, to gain permission from her father and the school for her to go to the UK. I set about investigating the possibility and making the case on the basis of her wellbeing. The doors opened in all of these avenues, and we planned our two-month trip.

The journey from thereon was eventful. We had a precarious flight heading to Wellington, with severe turbulence and the pilot aborted two landings which resulted in us going to Christchurch. My daughter was very calm through it all. She turned to me and said, "It's all right Mum, this pilot will have lots of experience." Passengers were vomiting, holding their hearts, and the facial expressions of the cabin crew concerned me. Thankfully we landed safely. Once we had sorted our connecting flight in Christchurch to Singapore, we decided to try and find the pilot to say thank you for getting us on the ground safely. We luckily found the cabin crew and pilot having breakfast together in the food court and we were able to thank him. He told us it was the worst turbulence he had encountered in his ten years of flying experience. My brain was ticking over thinking my cool-as-a-cucumber daughter coped admirably through this turbulence. I wondered if she had the makings of a pilot within her.

Fabulously, after this point we had great flight experiences, especially for Emily. Our flight from Christchurch to Singapore was practically empty and so we managed to sleep across vacant seats. The flight from Singapore to Heathrow was novel as our seats were upstairs at the very back, with extra leg room. Once in the UK, my sister had arranged with a friend who was a Cessna pilot to fly us from Oxford to Beverley. This was near where my mum lived, and we surprised her by arriving two weeks early. Emily sat in front of the Cessna and thoroughly enjoyed the experience.

The catalogue of experiences continued with the opportunity to go gliding over York. Shortly after getting out of the glider, Emily said with absolute certainty that she wanted to be a pilot. When back in New Zealand, she did her research about gaining a private pilot licence and the rest is history. She worked in the local fish and chip shop to help pay for the lessons, along with help from me and her dad. She got her private pilot licence at sixteen years of age for goodness sake! She applied to flight school to do her commercial flying course and got accepted, passed and graduated. She then trained as a flight instructor. She taught flight students and now works in the tourism industry, flying planes to boost her flight hours for her goal of flying for Air New Zealand.

This is a significant story. She is now 23 years of age. All of this transpired with her knowing what she needed. She followed up with stating clearly what she needed, then asking the question of whether her need could be met. Whether it was a big ask or not, she had the courage and valued herself enough to ask. The doors opened for us to follow this through. Her needs were met by spending time with her grandparents, and the inspirational flying experiences led to a purposeful direction in her life. I sometimes wonder would she have found this path that she loves with a passion if she hadn't asked for what she needed right back then? Would she have found it later? Possibly. The fact is that she asked, and she got more than what she asked for. I remember asking her if she had ever considered whether she would be flying planes if her father and I hadn't separated? There is always a silver lining somewhere.

I have to say that this was a lesson. I was not good at asking. I was also not good at receiving. I felt that I needed to handle everything and be coping. In fact, I was harsh with myself. I believed there was shame in asking for help. What I needed was gentleness and compassion towards myself. Possibly a lesson for us all. We need to stop for a minute and breathe to be aware of what we need. Support and self-care can lead to many great things.

An Ode of Compassion

This book is written warmly and with an appreciation for the varied journeys of solo mums. You may not know how awesome you are, perhaps because you are so busy and exhausted. Understandably so! According to Birthright New Zealand, 20% of families in New Zealand consist of single parents.

As a solo mum with no family in New Zealand, I know of the many pressures and responsibilities, and not knowing where to turn sometimes. Even with great friends around me the challenges were large. I felt like the mountain was very steep to climb, particularly regarding financial and emotional distress. Of course, the reasons for being in this position can differ in circumstances and dynamics. As you will have gathered, for me it was a divorce that catapulted us into this life-changing situation. Some solo parents may be caring for children (and adults) with disabilities or the challenges of neurodiversity. Some parents may be neurodiverse themselves, or experience a multitude of personal challenges. I suffered from dyscalculia and other cognitive traits on the spectrum that had never been diagnosed. This made looking at detailed small print, legal terms, working out the math of the divorce settlement, etc. very stressful.

The responsibilities and difficulties I remember seemed to be occurring simultaneously to begin with. I was literally trying to put one foot in front of the other, feeling completely overwhelmed on all levels, processing grief of separation/divorce while trying to hold it all together. Supporting and holding the space for my daughter to grieve the change in family circumstances; dealing with lawyers; feeling alone with decision making; self-doubt; low confidence; financial distress; job hunting; guilt of whether I was good enough to nurture my daughter on my own; worries that I might miss something that was crucial in keeping my daughter on her track; moving house (we moved four times in two years); car maintenance; house repairs; house and garden maintenance; managing work; and any prior trauma on top of it all. For some there may be bereavement through death of a beloved partner and dealing with the devastation associated with this. For whatever the reason, we try and be the rock.

The cumulative effect of soldiering on and forgetting that we need a break because we are so busy juggling many responsibilities leads us to high levels of stress, tiredness, and exhaustion that affects us physically, emotionally and mentally, subsequently impacting the spirit.

I remember having so many items on my to-do list that I was overwhelmed and couldn't prioritise them well. A friend/mentor suggested I have multiple lists. I constructed a list with seven columns at one point with different 'To Do' headings. The headings included Bills, School Activities, Work, Job Hunting, Football, House Hunting, Lawyer, Food Shopping and Housework/Chores. The lists were so helpful. I checked the list before going to sleep and added to it. The list gave me peace of mind that I had not forgotten anything, and it helped me to sleep! Hallelujah for the lists!! The beloved list became the glue that held my life together – my life support in keeping life on track, not missing a trick.

As time went by, I noticed that the emotional distress of the break-up was affecting my cognitive function, and it was noticeable at work. I felt shaky a lot of the time and I struggled to concentrate. I had a short attention span, I struggled to follow the flow of meetings, and my processing was slow. If it was happening at work, it must have been showing at home too. The realisation dawned on me that there was no column section on the list table for Jo-Anne. Despite my occupational therapy experience and Healing Touch training teaching me the importance of self-care, I still struggled to go beyond the pressure of the perceived essentials of the list. I was not walking the talk. That needed to change ... and I did.

As daughters, women, mothers and grandmothers, we deserve our self-care in our own right. As solo mums wanting to be the rock, the protector, the nurturer, we need to take our self-care diligently and luxuriously! Luxuriously can mean I am going to have that hot chocolate now and yes with four marshmallows. Or it could mean a ten-minute tea meditation ... whatever takes the mood! It doesn't have to break the bank.

There is an internal voice that creeps in – "The world will fall apart if you take your focus off the other things on the list", "You can't possibly take your eye off the ball for more than five minutes", "What if she needs you and you aren't there ..." Well, how interesting that not taking enough self-care did in fact contribute to not being able to focus and concentrate on the ball very well at all.

The purpose of *Solo Mums Matter* is to support and encourage restoration, relaxation, to raise the spirit, bringing enjoyment and an increase in your energy levels. During the process we can reconnect with personal purpose and direction. This book aims to prevent or turn around common self-neglect, prevent or break the cumulative cycle of stress, fatigue/exhaustion and per-ceived barriers to self-care, and provide accessible tools. It brings together my time as an occupational therapist, a Dancing Way instructor, Healing Touch practitioner and experience in designing and running fatigue management groups.

At the end of the day, we know that when we look after ourselves and our energy levels, a ripple effect is felt. We feel good, everything seems to flow better, answers to problems seem to come more easily and we enjoy life more. Ultimately this has a positive effect on our relationships with ourselves, family, friends, work colleagues, etc. It seems simple on paper. The realities make it harder to break our patterns and burst through our blockages. As solo mums we can do it. We need to be self-compassionate for ourselves physically, emotionally, mentally/cognitively, and spiritually. We are present. Women and mums on our game! We don't always get it right, but we can aim for some balance and restoration.

I would like to make a short note on affirmations. Affirmations are useful. However, don't be tempted to use them as a method of stuffing emotions down. Feelings and emotions that may be deemed as negative do need expression in a safe way. This was brought to my attention when I was receiving psycho-synthesis therapy. I found this to be great advice. Affirmations are helpful to bring to your conscious mind the positive changes that you would like to make in your life alongside the expression of grief, letting the tears roll and feeling righteous anger. Tears are healing and cleansing, creating a space for moving forwards. Expression of anger safely can also help movement forwards.

How to Use This Book

I ask you to follow what resonates with you personally. One thing that I have learnt is that fatigue/energy management is an individual journey of self-care. While there are some things that will help all of us with increasing our energy levels, there are unique needs particular to you. There is no one-size-fits-all. That's why you can't prescribe in this work. It's your journey of finding what's right for you. Your needs are your personal needs, your wants are your personal wants, your dreams are your personal dreams. So, in these pages, you are indeed the focus in the context of your life.

1. These chapters are supportive companions. I recommend reading a chapter a week or over a few weeks. Make a pact to read the chapters, even if in short bursts. Try the taster activities, tools and strategies so that you know what resonates. I have made most of the activities short, energy-boosting and self-discovering. Making a commitment to yourself means that you value *you*. It may be that first thing in the morning, or last thing at night, when the kids are at school or at football practice, etc. might be the best time to read or do an activity. Whatever the situation,

be gentle with yourself and pace yourself. Pushing through is not allowed. Rest when you need to. The chapters can take as long as you need.

2. I would recommend working through each chapter in sequential order, and to consistently start each chapter on a Sunday or a Monday – this way you can plan and schedule more easily.

3. Each chapter has a treasury of information, taster activities, tools and strategies, journalling to find your personal energy tonics. This is all for information-gathering and moving forwards. After reading a chapter, scan through the taster activities, tools and strategies so that you can decide which to select first, and it will help you to plan your week/s.

4. As you move through each chapter, you may identify that you need extra support. Chapter Nine has a list of supportive organisations which offer a variety of support, guidance and resources. Be sure to check out this chapter if your needs/signposts are indicating that extra help is needed. Also please ensure that if you identify a medical health need, you arrange an appointment as part of your self-care.

5. Resonance is a concept that really relates to the heart. *The American Heritage Dictionary of the English Language* (online, 2024) defines to resonate as 'to correspond closely or harmoniously'. It feels like something rings true for you and may even make your heart sing. So, when scanning through the taster activities, tools and strategies, see what resonates with you to try first. Take note of what works for you, how you feel regarding your energy levels and your fatigue sign severity. Be aware of any activities that you don't like the sound of and take note of these, asking yourself why you aren't keen. Aim to do them all and then you can cross off the list in terms of which is a no, or a resounding yes. Discernment is key in establishing what is going to be restorative and relaxing. *The American Heritage Dictionary of the English Language* defines discernment for us as being 'keenness of insight and judgment'.

6. I recommend journalling for many reasons. It can be useful in getting down onto the pages your feelings, thoughts, emotions, reflections, making sense of things and writing your story – a great process of acknowledging, validating, releasing and letting go. It's private between you, your pen and the journal. For me, my journal was my private therapy where I could safely express the range of emotions I was going through. I could use whatever language I liked and make holes in the paper with the pen if I felt angry!! No guilt! Don't let anyone tell you that anger is wrong. How we use it is what counts.

    Anger is another helpful signpost if we can decipher the message it is trying to signal. Make sense of it on the page. When all is calm, act on the message to resolve things and move forwards. I have a story on that one later. Let it spill onto the page … let it run its course. One of the temptations is to discuss our personal difficulties, relationships, etc. with our children and overshare. Get it onto the page instead; the page is another loyal ally. When we write in the journal, we have the opportunity to compassionately tell our truth from our perspective.

    Julia Cameron, in her book *The Artist's Way*, advocates doing 'morning pages' upon waking – three pages of just writing anything. It doesn't matter what you write, the purpose is to start clearing and unblocking. Interesting nuggets of information can start to drop out of the pages. Committing to every morning might be a challenge depending on your circumstances and how young your children are. I did my journalling when it arose as a need, as well as most nights. It helped solve some problems with great light-bulb moments. If you feel that you need a bit of extra help, e.g. counselling, explore Chapter Nine for some of the options and organisations who can guide and support.

7. Chapter One describes fatigue and lists numerous fatigue signs to increase awareness. This can be confronting; pace yourself if needed. Tick the boxes which apply to you and then relax into the exercises. The exercises are exploratory and immediately introduce you to strategies to begin breaking the cycle of fatigue.

8. From Chapter One onwards you are encouraged to engage in an enjoyable activity that is just for *you* alone. Not with the children or *for* the children … for *you*. Fun stuff with the kids is classed as separate activities.

9. In some of the taster activities, tools and strategies, there are 'attention to breathing' exercises. Some people prefer to gently read them closing their eyes between each section or line of the scripts. It may also be useful to record your voice saying the script so that your voice can be your guide through the exercise.

Serenity Prayer

I feel it poignant at this point to recognise those 'things', circumstances or people that cannot be changed. We ourselves instead can grow and a positive ripple effect can be felt for ourselves and others. With our hearts open and taking courageous steps, doors naturally open. I came across this serenity prayer by Reinhold Niebuhr on three separate occasions in the space of a month. I take it as a nudge to include it in this book. If it resonates with you, refer to this serenity prayer and say it out loud when you feel the need.

"God, grant me the serenity
to accept the things I cannot change,
the courage to change the things I can,
and the wisdom to know the difference."

Commitment Agreement

I .... *Your Name* .... agree to take steps to be
compassionate and gentle with myself while progressing
through these pages, taster activities, tools and strategies. I
commit to pacing myself according to my energy needs and
responding to my fatigue signs in the process of restoring.

.... *Your Signature* ....

References

1. *The American Heritage Dictionary of the English Language*, Definition of 'discernment'. Available at: https://ahdictionary.com/word/search.html?q=discernment (Accessed: September 2024).
2. *The American Heritage Dictionary of the English Language*, Definition of 'resonates'. Available at: https://ahdictionary.com/word/search.html?q=resonates (Accessed: September 2024).

CHAPTER ONE

A Treasury of Fatigue Awareness and Self-Compassion

Fatigue is a word that is used widely, but it isn't attributed to just standard tiredness. There are many conditions which exhibit fatigue symptoms. What is relevant is that solo mums are prone to burnout and compassion fatigue. Compassion fatigue can include emotional, physical and spiritual distress in those caring for another. As mums, we are caring for the physical, emotional, mental and spiritual needs of the family. Life can feel intense on all levels, and we empathetically give to meet the needs of family as well as trying to keep everything ticking over. We need to be empathetic to ourselves so that we have empathy for our kids.

Compassion fatigue is a common diagnosis for health professionals working intensely with others' needs on all of these levels and single mums are a prime candidate for experiencing this. From a burnout perspective this is a state of emotional, mental and physical exhaustion caused by prolonged stress, overwork and lack of balance in life. So as solo mums, we can be prone to this also. I would say that the two of these are connected.

When we experience too many pressures and too much emotional, physical and mental fatigue for too long, exhaustion sets in. Energy is depleted with no more left in the tank to give. It's time to acknowledge that something needs to change and begin to receive so that we can restore ourselves!

The Compassion Fatigue Awareness Project (2024) which is available to view online, emphasises that 'accepting the presence of compassion fatigue in our lives only serves to validate the fact that we are deeply caring individuals … It is possible to practice healthy, ongoing self-care while successfully caring for others'.

The symptoms of compassions fatigue and burnout are signs of high levels of stress. In today's living, most of us have high levels of cortisol in our bodies due to stress which contribute to many problems including adrenal fatigue. We can reduce this.

Often, we are taught to care for the needs of others before our own needs. Over a prolonged period, we realise that we can't sustain this. Some of us try even harder if it's in our nature.

If this resonates with you then you can choose to embark on a journey of discovery for YOU to YOU. You will be guided to an awareness of patterns and traits, where they may stem from, move through the barriers in order that you can give yourself what you need, or be able to ask for what you need. Gentleness with yourself is paramount. What we are in fact looking to nurture is self-compassion.

Self-compassion is the ability to recognise when you are being harsh with yourself and replace harshness with gentleness and kindness. Self-compassion is knowing and responding gently to the fact that humans struggle and suffer sometimes. Self-compassion is identifying a self-care need and allowing for those needs to be met. It's like being your own best friend or treating yourself like a great friend. Neff (2024), in an online article titled 'What is Self- Compassion?' states that self-compassion means being supportive when you're facing a life challenge, feel inadequate, or make a mistake. Instead of just ignoring your pain with a stiff upper lip mentality or getting carried away by your negative thoughts and emotions, you stop to tell yourself, "This is really difficult right now, how can I comfort and care for myself in this moment?" Instead of mercilessly judging and criticising yourself for various inadequacies or shortcomings, self-compassion means you are kind and understanding when confronted with your failings – after all, who ever said you were supposed to be perfect? Neff maintains that there are three main elements of compassion: mindfulness, common humanity, and kindness.

The Cumulative Effects of Fatigue

The cumulative signs of fatigue can affect us physically, emotionally, mentally, spiritually and behaviourally. They are all interconnected and affect each other.

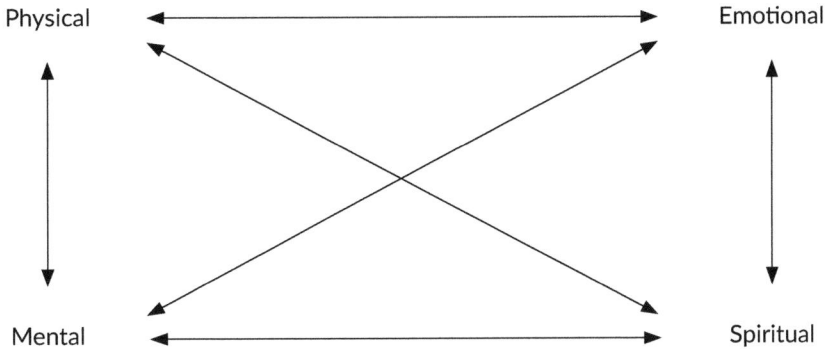

For example, say your child wants to ask you something about their homework. You've had a challenging day with no tea breaks or lunch and feel frazzled and drained. At work that afternoon you were unable to focus on the computer screen or follow what was going on in the meeting. You feel that you need to help with your child's homework so you say, "Yep, how can I help?" Your child starts explaining and you are struggling to listen and concentrate to make sense of the question. You ask your child to explain the question again and you still haven't got it. You start to feel frustrated with yourself, you can hear the negative self-talk and the internal upset escalating. Your child is starting to feel frustrated. You squash down the upset and say, "Okay, I will make myself a cup of tea and we will try again in 20 minutes." You are feeling full of emotion and on the way into the kitchen you lose your sense of awareness in space and knock your shoulder on the doorframe. It all comes flooding out, the tears and frustration.

Looking at it with hindsight, this cycle could've been broken. You would've taken rest breaks and lunch at work. If the boss said he needed that report by 2 pm, you would have said that you needed your break first. You were more likely to have met the deadline as you feel more productive having taken the breaks. If the kettle went on as soon as you got home and you took a well-needed 20 minutes out, I wonder how the homework scenario would play out? The cumulative effect of fatigue can snowball for days, weeks, months and years until we can't continue any longer in the same way. You then have no choice but to take a huge break. The knack is breaking the cycle early. The following adage is relevant, that we can't keep pouring water from the glass unless we take regular pauses to keep refilling it. The feeling of exhaustion will magnify, and we are halted.

I have listed some fatigue signs below. Put a tick beside any that you experience regularly. You can really understand how we can feel in an absolute quagmire of sensations and difficulties when you look at the list of possible ways people can be affected. Some of your signs may come and go and sometimes they can feel as if they appear all at the same time.

Be gentle with yourself here. We are establishing where you are at so that you can gently move forwards in a self-caring way, a bit at a time and recognise when you need to stop and take a break. Making small adjustments to your self-care routine can make a huge difference in how you can manage the symptoms you may identify below. These signs really are your allies and have a purpose as signposts alerting you to your self-care needs. They are showing you that something needs to change and setting boundaries for yourself is required for your needs to be met. Your awareness is a very positive stage. It may seem confronting, uncomfortable and overwhelming as you see the overall picture. It is the first step of breaking the cumulative cycle of fatigue.

Physical Effects
- Muscular fatigue
- Aches and pains
- Slow movement
- Difficult to coordinate movement
- Balance difficulties
- Slower response times
- Dizziness
- Headaches
- Migraines

- Slurred speech
- Unclear communication, possibly jumbled up
- Nausea
- Sleepiness and struggling to keep eyes open
- Frequent yawning
- Struggle to actively listen/hear
- Increase in accidents and injuries
- Other

Emotional Effects
- Feeling of overwhelm
- Feeling not able to cope
- Feeling unhappy
- Increase in blaming
- Increase in complaining
- Loneliness
- Frustration
- Irritability
- Anger
- Worry
- Stress
- Anxiety
- Guilt
- Grief
- Crying a lot
- Suppression of emotion
- Less communicative/quieter
- Concern about what other might think
- Other

Mental Effects
- Reduced ability to concentrate
- Foggy feeling and unable to think

- ☆ Slower processing of information
- ☆ Reduced awareness of difficulties
- ☆ Difficulties reasoning
- ☆ Difficulties problem solving
- ☆ Difficulties learning new information
- ☆ Difficulties remembering
- ☆ Difficulties word finding
- ☆ Difficulties making choices
- ☆ Difficulties with making decisions
- ☆ Reduced awareness of self, others and the environment
- ☆ Think you are inadequate
- ☆ Think you are unworthy
- ☆ Think you are lazy or negative self-talk if take a rest
- ☆ Other

Spiritual Effects

- ☆ Zoning out
- ☆ Feeling spaced out like you aren't fully present
- ☆ Loss of sense of meaning to life
- ☆ Loss of sense of personal purpose
- ☆ Loss of sense of enjoyment
- ☆ Loss of that spark that makes your heart sing
- ☆ Loss of sense of autonomy
- ☆ Feeling that everything is automated and on autopilot
- ☆ Reduction in motivation
- ☆ Other

Behavioural Effects

- ☆ Cut corners
- ☆ Make more mistakes
- ☆ Try harder, driven by internal expectations (high self-expectations)
- ☆ Driven by external expectations, e.g. to please others
- ☆ Push yourself harder despite the fatigue

- Withdraw from friends
- Withdraw from socialising
- Withdraw from family
- Other

Typical Causes of Fatigue

- High expectations of yourself
- People-pleasing
- Traits, e.g. a natural empathetic person
- Traits, e.g. perfectionism
- Traits, e.g. workaholism
- Fear of perceived failure
- Unhealthy habits re alcohol/substances
- Very full routines
- Stress
- Self-neglect – no self-care
- Fear of being seen to be not coping so reluctant to ask or accept help
- Suppression of emotion
- Difficulties asking for help
- Difficulties receiving help
- Shallow breathing
- Not enough quality sleep
- Poor diet
- Dehydration
- Toxicity
- Weakened immune system
- Overstretching boundaries
- Inability to say no when you need to and want to
- Difficulties setting boundaries, i.e. creating time and space for needs to be met
- Disconnect from sensations in our bodies and therefore can't respond to needs

✿   Boom-and-bust approach to tasks, e.g. can't stop until completed tasks and then crash

✿   Lack of exercise

✿   Lack of interests and hobbies

✿   Negative views around resting

✿   Imbalance of giving and receiving

✿   Environment, e.g. cold, hot, loud, lighting, electromagnetic sensitivity

✿   Other

Take note of the category areas where your fatigue may show up more, e.g. physically, emotionally, mentally and spiritually. It may be that you have a scattering across these aspects. Also take note of traits, behaviours, routines and other causes that may resonate with you.

Triggers

You may notice that there are certain times of the day, times of the week or month where the fatigue signs appear or are more magnified. Take note of these. Also take note of the environment, who you are with, and what you are doing. See if you notice any signs that emerge in certain situations. It will be important for you to know. Keep notes in your journal.

TASTER ACTIVITIES, TOOLS AND STRATEGIES

1.   **Self-Compassion Meditation (approx. 20 minutes)**
     a.   Make yourself comfortable in a supportive chair, with your feet flat on the ground, your spine as straight as possible and your hands resting in your lap.
     b.   Knowing that you are supported by the chair and the ground, pay attention to the pathway of your breath. In through your nose and out through your nose …

c. Without trying to change the way that you are breathing at all, just notice your natural rhythm of breathing …

d. If you hear sounds around you, just let them pass through …

e. Settle in to being aware of your breathing pattern … notice the rise and fall of your chest …

f. Notice the slight gentle rise and fall of your tummy area …

g. Take your focus to your heart area as you breathe …

h. Imagine that your heart is filling with the colour of golden pink as you breathe in, feel warmth in your heart area, and then breathe out tension. Repeat for four cycles of breath.

i. Feel the relaxation and gentleness of your heart.

j. Feel a loving acceptance and kindness for who you are in this moment … feel the love and compassion that you have for yourself.

k. The tension is melting away with each in and out breath.

l. Feel the presence of unconditional love in your heart.

m. Let your unconditional love flow from your heart into every cell of your body …

n. Enjoy the feeling of bathing in unconditional love …

o. You know that you can choose to be in unconditional love with yourself … be present with the feeling of unconditional love.

p. When you are ready, bring your awareness back to your breathing, feel your feet on the ground, the backs of your legs on the seat and being supported by the chair …

q. Sit quietly for a short while to orientate … take self-compassion and unconditional love into the next phase of your day.

2. **Box Breathing (5 minutes)**

A powerful but simple relaxation technique that aims to return breathing to its usual rhythm if feeling stressed. Navy SEALs use this technique to relieve stress and remedy shallow breathing. It can help clear the mind, relax the body, recentre and improve concentration. When box breathing you are activating the parasympathetic nervous system. This is the rest-and-digest mode, rather than the fight-or-flight mode of the sympathetic nervous system. You can do this anywhere (not while driving). You can think of a box as you are breathing if you like.

a. Breathe out slowly, releasing all the air from your lungs.

b. Breathe in through your nose, counting in your head to four slowly, feeling the air entering your lungs.

c. Hold your breath for a count of four.

d. Exhale for a count of four.

e. Hold your breath again for a count of four.

f. Repeat all of the above for three to four rounds.

3. **Breathing with Awareness and Body Scan (approx. 30 minutes or for as long as you like)**

a. Make yourself comfortable in a supportive chair, with your feet flat on the ground, your spine as straight as possible and your hands resting in your lap.

b. Knowing that you are supported by the chair and the ground, pay attention to the pathway of your breath, in through your nose and out through your nose.

c. Without trying to change the way that you are breathing at all, just notice your natural rhythm of breathing.

d. If you hear sounds around you, just let them pass through.

e. Settle in to being aware of your breathing.

f. If your mind wanders, bring your focus back to your breathing.

g. Notice the gentle rising and falling of your chest as you breathe.

h. Notice the slight gentle rise and fall of your tummy area as you breathe.

i. Turn your focus to your feet. Notice any sensation in your toes or the soles of your feet. Imagine each in breath flowing to your feet. On each exhale let go of tension from your feet.

j. Move your attention to your ankles and calf muscles. Notice any tension that you may be holding there. Notice how the muscles feel here. With each in and out breath feel the muscles softening.

k. Your thighs are being supported by the chair. How are they feeling? Allow them to feel heavier on each out breath. Your knees and hips, how are they being held ... are they restful? Allow the joints and muscles to simply be.

l. Pay attention to how your lower back feels ... then your abdomen ... upper back ... chest ... shoulders ... arms ... hands ... notice where any tension is being held ...

m. Focus on your stomach gently rising and falling as you breathe ... letting go. Notice movement in your chest area as you breathe ... letting go.

n. Now imagine that from the base of your skull there is a gentle warm flow of water running over your neck ... your shoulders ... and down your back ... washing away any tension that you may have there. You find the warmth of the water soothing, comforting and deeply relaxing. The water gently washes over your shoulders and down your arms to your hands and fingertips. Tension is being washed away.

o. Feet relaxed, legs relaxed, front of the body relaxed, back of the body relaxed, shoulders, arms, hands, fingers relaxed, neck is now relaxed. Notice how your jaw is held ... is there a gap between your teeth ... or are they clenching. Allow the muscles around your jaw to soften ... how does your tongue feel ... allow it to rest gently behind your teeth.

p. Allow the skin over your cheekbones to soften and relax.

q. Your eyes resting in their sockets behind your eyelids ... feel them relaxing ... peaceful.

r. Notice any frown on your forehead ... smooth away any frown that you may have there ... smoothing out your forehead.

s. Relaxing through your ears.

t. Your scalp softening.

u. Steadily do a scan through your body ... if you sense any tension ... breathe into it giving yourself permission to let it go.

v. Start to become aware of your surroundings in this room ... hear the sounds, feel your feet on the ground, move a part of your body that wants to move ... stretch ... yawn or sigh ... sit quietly for a short while to reorientate.

4. **Self-Care Activities (20 minutes)**

   Write two lists in your journal. The first list being what you do to self-care. The second list being what leisure activities you engage in. If you aren't engaging much in self-care or leisure activities don't worry, think of times when you have and list those.

5. **Life Balance (30 minutes)**

   Turner (2002) states that activities are the means through which people control the balance in their lives ... People make decisions about what they will and won't do and when, where, how and with whom they will do it.

   Consider the number of hours that you spend on the areas of life below. Do this for a typical weekday and a weekend day. Leisure may be a mix of spending time on your own during leisure activities, or with your family. Productivity/work could be any paid work, household chores and paying the bills, etc.

   Weekday

Rest/Sleep	_____ hours
Self-Care	_____ hours
Leisure	_____ hours
Productivity/Work	_____ hours

   Weekend Day

Rest/Sleep	_____ hours
Self-Care	_____ hours
Leisure	_____ hours
Productivity/Work	_____ hours

   We will refer to this activity in the following chapters.

6.   **Clearing Space: Room for You! (45 minutes)**

Clearing out items that no longer resonate with you, or that you don't need any more, is synonymous with creating space for something new in your life.

- Find a large cardboard box and place it somewhere that's easily accessible, but not in the way.
- As you go about the day around home, start looking at things through a lens of whether it is functional, are you likely to use it, does it bring you enjoyment, do you still like it or want it.
- If the answer is no to any of these questions, then put it in the box.
- Once in the box, resist the temptation of taking it back out of the box.
- The filling of the box can be done gradually during the next few weeks.
- After two weeks, take it to the op shop and feel the lightness of letting go.

7.   **An Enjoyable Artistic Pursuit (30 minutes or more)**

This does not have to be a major production of art! It could be as simple as putting your favourite music on and dancing, or painting to the rhythm of the music. Whatever suits you. Just because you can. If you think it's silly that's okay, you have a licence to be silly. Art doesn't have to be serious, but it **can** be if you want it to. It just must be enjoyable and arty. This is about letting go! Think back over the years to the enjoyable art pursuits that you did as a kid, teenager, adult. List five of your enjoyable pursuits.

1._____

2._____

3._____

4._____

5._____

Choose one and enjoy doing it ... just for the fun and love of it! There is one rule – it's **your** time. See if you can find a quiet slot for just you.

8.   Journal Suggestions

- Write down in your journal any thoughts or feelings about your findings so far, and anything that is happening for you in general.
- Which taster activities, tools and strategies worked well for you?
- Did anything stand out and how did you feel?
- Do you feel that any of the information, taster activities, tools and strategies will help reduce your fatigue signs?
- Have you noticed any changes in your fatigue signs, their severity and your energy levels?
- You may feel that you want to monitor your energy levels and fatigue signs. You can do this by regularly checking in with how you are feeling during certain activities and in different environments. There may even be a link with your energy levels/signs and certain places/activities.

9.   My Personal Energy Tonic Treasury (20 minutes)

In your journal draw your discerning resonant heart as shown below. It may need to take up the full page.

INNER HEART

- Write in the inner heart the points that have strongly stood out and resonated in the treasury of information, taster activities/ strategies/ tools that you want to include in your daily life **straight away**.
- Reflect on whether these things have been helpful towards reducing your fatigue signs and increasing your energy levels.
- Consult your journal and transfer anything else that is important to you. This may include the adapting or letting go of certain activities or routines, etc. that you have realised drain you of energy. It could also include ways that you can pace certain activities.

OUTER HEART

- Write in the outer heart the things you have identified that resonate with you and that you would like to change or include in your life **at some point in the future**.

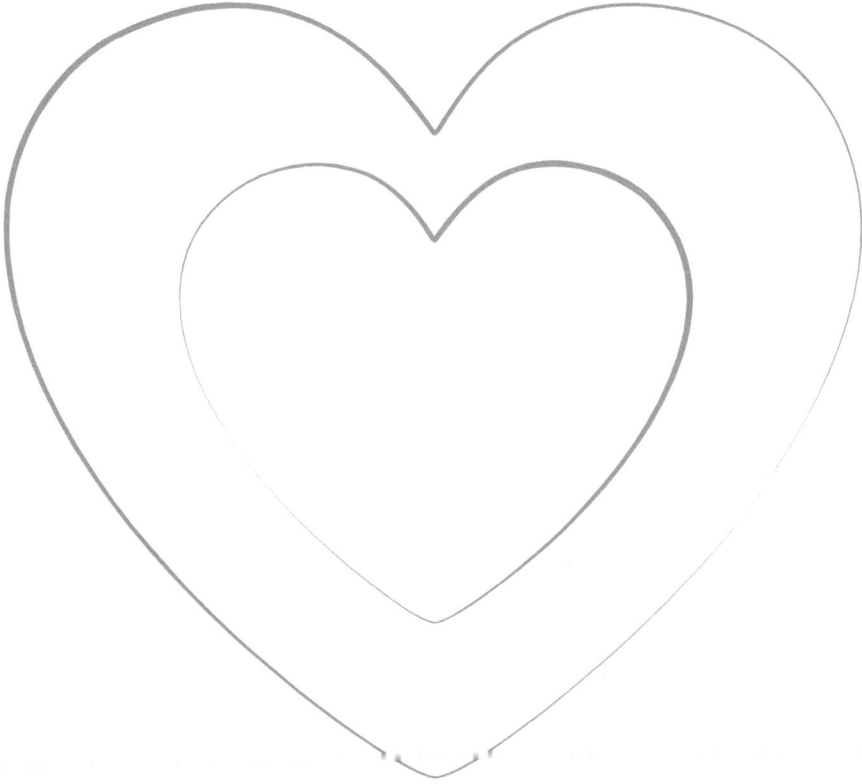

Congratulations! You have dedicated at least three hours and 20 minutes towards restoring your energy levels through these energy taster activities, tools and strategies. This doesn't include your journalling time.

References

1. Compassion Fatigue Awareness Project. Available at: https://compassionfatigue.org/index.html (Accessed September 2024).
2. Neff, K., Dr. *What is Self-Compassion?* Available at: https://self-compassion.org/what-is-self-compassion/ (Accessed October 2024).
3. Turner, A., TDipCOT MA FCOT (2002) Foster, M.A. and Johnson, S.E. *Occupational Therapy and Physical Dysfunction: Principles, Skills and Practice*, 5e. 5 Edition. Churchill Livingstone.

CHAPTER TWO

A Treasury of Life Energy

It's useful to understand how energy works within your body when looking at self-care choices and the various ways of increasing energy levels. This is a huge topic, and you may want to follow up with further reading on some of the threads described here. When everything is looked at under a microscope, the whole process of life is energetic. Everything from unseen energy to what exists as matter in the physical form is a vibration of energy. I have opted to take a holistic approach to provide a broad perspective. Whether you realise it or not, life is in fact an energy game, and we need to adapt how we play the game as life changes. Discern what resonates with you, because you are your own player.

The Self-Perpetuating Human Body

Marieb (1989) in 'Chemistry Comes Alive' states that all living things are composed as matter and, to grow and function, they all require energy. It is the release and use of the energy in human systems that give us the elusive quality called life.

Life is an indication of energy within the body, and Chang (1986) explains the human body as a 'self-perpetuating human body', like a battery. The human battery can be described as having three 'vital parts'.

- Structure: the cells and the organs, bones, muscle, skin layers, blood vessels, nerves and other physical structures that they form.
- Liquid: the intracellular and intercellular liquids that play important roles in the generation of electrical energy.
- Electrical charge: the charge that is responsible for activating the body and its structures. It is called 'life force', 'life energy', 'spirit', 'electromagnetism', 'chi'.

To describe how this works we will look at structure in terms of the function of mitochondria within the cells. For liquid we will look at water. For the electrical charge we will look at electromagnetic energy, the human energy anatomy including the human biofield, energy centres and pathways.

Vital Part: Structure
Mitochondria in Energy Production

There are energy factory structures within our cells called mitochondria. In the mitochondria, food is turned into the currency of cellular energy called ATP (Adenosine Tri Phosphate). This process also needs oxygen. The more ATP that is produced, the more energy the cell will have. It is therefore important that we have healthy mitochondria if these are the sites for our energy production.

A Metagenics Seminar titled 'Energy for Life, Natural Approaches to the Treatment of Fatigue,' lists these factors as impactors on mitochondrial function:

- Stress
- Infection
- Metabolism
- Inflammation
- Toxicity
- Poor nutrition

This suggests that our physical, emotional, mental and spiritual wellbeing affects energy production at a cellular level. In the business of life juggling, we can easily forget about these aspects of ourselves. Our awareness may be drowned out under pressure. On autopilot we don't respond.

Also, it is important to realise that every single bodily system, e.g. the circulatory system, digestive system, renal system, nervous system and associated organs have a role in processing and enabling the delivery of energy or eliminating waste. These systems keep energy supplies flowing to maintain life. Each of these systems are regenerated with new cells which also requires energy from the mitochondria. These energy factories, in every single cell within every system of the body, serve to respond with an energy-production balancing act to maintain and sustain life. What an intricate design that deserves respect! This system asks or tells us what it needs so that we can contribute to it working effectively. It can be as simple as responding to the sensation of hunger and taking a break to eat.

All of this is significant food for thought as we think about the ways we can help support mitochondrial function. It also brings home the fact that everything we choose to do has a direct influence on our energy. Some specific positive ways to support our energy levels will be highlighted in this and the following chapters.

Vital Part: Liquid
Water in Energy Production

Water is mainly obtained from ingested foods or liquids and is lost from the body by exhaling, through the skin and excreted by the kidneys. Human survival is of course dependent on it, and we are literally water. The cells and the organs, bones, muscle, skin layers, blood vessels, nerves and other physical structures that they form all require water. The mitochondria require water with its oxygen content to make ATP the energy currency.

Marieb (1989) states that water is the most abundant and important inorganic compound found in living material, making up from around 60–80% of the volume of most living cells. The versatility of this vital fluid is incredible … It provides the liquid environment necessary for chemical reactions …

Dorchester Health (2014) says that the human body is a water machine, designed to run on water and minerals. Every life-giving and healing process that happens inside our body … happens with water … The human body is made up of over 70% water. Our blood is more than 80%, our brain over 75% and the human liver is an amazing 96% water … Our energy level is greatly affected by the amount of water we drink. It has been medically proven that just a 5% drop in body fluids will cause a 25% to 30% loss of energy in the average person … Water is what our liver uses to metabolise fat into useable energy. It is estimated that over 80% of the population suffers energy loss due to minor dehydration.

- Water is the medium for various enzymatic and chemical reactions in the body. It moves nutrients, hormones, antibodies and oxygen through the blood stream and lymphatic system. The proteins and the enzymes of the body function more efficiently in solutions of lower viscosity. Water is the solvent of the body, and it regulates all functions, including the activity of everything it dissolves and circulates.
- Water helps regulate our body temperature through perspiration, which dissipates excess heat and cools our bodies.
- We even need water to breathe. As we take in oxygen, we excrete CO_2; our lungs must be moistened by water. We lose up to two pints of water each day just by exhaling.
- The kidneys remove wastes such as uric acid, urea and lactic acid, all of which must be dissolved in water. When there isn't sufficient water, those wastes are not effectively removed which may result in damage to the kidneys.
- Water lubricates our joints. The cartilage tissues found at the end of the long bones and between the vertebrae of the spine hold a lot of water, which serves as a lubricant during the movement of the joint. When the cartilage is well hydrated, the two opposing surfaces glide freely, and friction damage is minimal. If the cartilage is dehydrated, the rate

of abrasive damage is increased, resulting in joint deterioration and increased pain.

☆ The actively growing blood cells in the bone marrow take priority over the cartilage for the available water that goes through the bone structure.

☆ Brain tissue is 85% water. Although the brain is only 1/50th of the body weight, it uses 1/20th of the blood supply. With dehydration, the level of energy generation in the brain is decreased. Depression and chronic fatigue syndrome are frequent results of dehydration.

Just to make a case in point and without going into too much detail, here are 14 energy processes that take place within the body requiring water:

1. Potential energy = stored energy within the cells
2. Chemical energy = stored in the chemical bonds, e.g. food
3. Kinetic energy = energy in action within the cells
4. Metabolism = all the chemical processes and energy changes needed for life, including anabolism and catabolism
5. Anabolism = synthesis or construction of molecules from smaller ones
6. Catabolism = breakdown of larger molecules into smaller ones
7. Basal metabolism = minimum energy needed to maintain life functions of the body, e.g. respiration, circulation
8. Cellular respiration = aerobic and anaerobic respiration
9. Aerobic respiration = requires oxygen to generate energy
10. Anaerobic respiration = occurs in the absence of oxygen
11. Electrical energy = cells and nervous system
12. Action potential = short-term change in the electrical potential to the surface of the cell, e.g. a nerve or muscle cell
13. Mechanical energy = leg movements to move a pedal on a bike
14. Homeostasis = the process through which the body adapts to maintain its equilibrium or balance

It is very clear that water is a fundamental requirement for energy processes within the body.

Vital Part: Electromagnetic Energy
The Biofield, Chakras and the Meridians

Chang (1986) explains that electromagnetism is an intensity force that permeates the atomic structures of all objects, including the surrounding atmosphere. Because it is a natural force, it has a rapport with the energy within the body.

Gimbel (2005), in the book *The Healing Energies of Colour*, describes that everything on earth takes in and releases energy. The process of life and growth involves the exchange of energy with the environment – an input and output. Part of the output is a unique energy field that exists around every living being, including human beings. Think of a human being as having not only the immediately visible physical body, but emanations of this subtle output energy that surrounds the body but are not visible (or only visible to some). They perform the protective zone of transition between the physical body and the outside world. This area is called an aura. It holds life energy and reflects the state of health … The layers of the aura have different colours and are related to different functions. The vibration and colours of the layers of a human aura alter as a result of internal changes in health and consciousness and the effects of the environment.

In terms of the electromagnetic aspects of the human body, Oschman (2009) poses that electrical conductivity in the body works from the surface of the skin inward to the organs inside the body. All are part of the full-body living matrix needed for the communication necessary for life and physical function.

Anderson et al. (2017) state that the human energy system can be viewed as numerous energy fields working in concert to maintain fundamental biological processes. These fields include the biofield surrounding the body, multiple local energy centres concentrated in specific areas of the body, and energetic pathways that regulate the flow of energy within the body. Each of these categories of energy fields correspond with energy systems described in the ancient health traditions of cultures worldwide. For example, the aura refers to the biofield, the chakras of Eastern cultures refer to the local energy centres located throughout the body, and the meridians of traditional Chinese medicine are the energetic pathways.

There are seven layers to the human biofield surrounding the body, with the outer layer forming an egg shape.

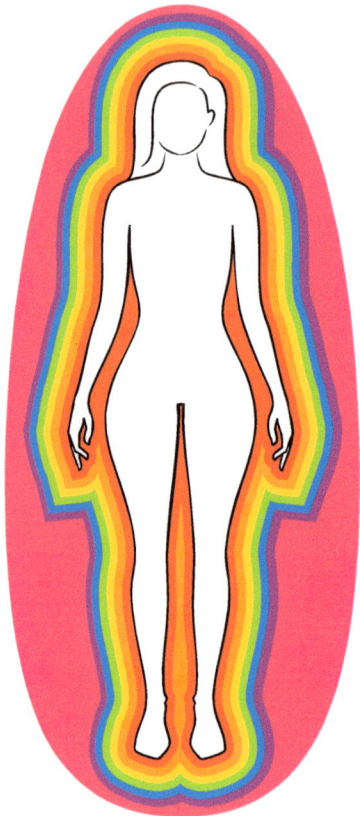

The layer closest to the physical body is the etheric layer

The second layer is the emotional layer

The third layer is the mental layer

The fourth layer is the spiritual layer

The fifth layer is the optimal blueprint of the physical body – the physical of the spiritual layers

The sixth layer is the emotional level of the spiritual layers

The seventh layer is the mental layer of the spiritual layers and forms the outer edge and boundary of the biofield

Karagulla et al. (1989) point out that the most important function of the etheric body is the transfer of life energy or vitality from the universal field to the individual field, and thence to the physical body. It is the primary contact with the ocean of life energy that sustains all of nature. Vitality is not recognised as a form of energy in the West, but in the East, where it is known as 'prana', it has always been perceived as a universal force in nature connected with breathing and breath. The etheric also acts as a connecting link between the physical body and the emotional and mental vehicles, although all of these are interpenetrating and synchronised, thus constituting the physical body, the instrument of the conscious self during the whole of life.

The second part of the human energy system is the chakra system (see page 36). Chakras are energy vortices that enable electromagnetic energy flow into the cells of the body. Each major chakra functions at a certain frequency which emanates a specific colour, relates to a particular endocrine gland, organ, musical note, relates to specific functions and psychological aspects. Healing Touch practitioners can assess the human energy field and chakra system. They work with intention and energy techniques to bring the energy system into balance. On a personal note, throughout the most stressful times in my, life Healing Touch has been a balm and a relief when I have felt under immense pressure and exhausted physically, emotionally and mentally. A gentle and relaxing modality of restoring energy balance and flow.

The third part of the energy system are the meridians as described in traditional Chinese medicine. The meridians work together in corresponding pairs that relate to an element in nature. The chart on page 37 shows the correspondences between the elements, the respective meridians, what they govern in terms of functions, sense organs and related sounds. It is believed that unexpressed grief may energetically block the air element meridians. Excessive fear can affect energy flow in the water element meridians. Suppression of anger can affect flow in the wood element channels and so forth.

Acupuncturists and shiatsu therapists work with the meridian system, as does the practice of tai chi. Acupuncturists and shiatsu practitioners work along the acupuncture points to balance or unblock energy flow. In the case of tai chi, gentle movement sequences engage energy flow through the meridians.

The meridian channels are in the bioenergy field. They connect with the chakras and direct energy flow up and down the body. Geddes et al. (1999) explain that each meridian passes partly through the body and partly along the skin, joining various chakras and organs. One end of each meridian is beneath the skin while the other is on the surface of the skin on the feet or hands. Along each meridian are acupressure points. These allow the flow of energy from the chakras and organs, and from the meridians with ends located on the feet and hands.

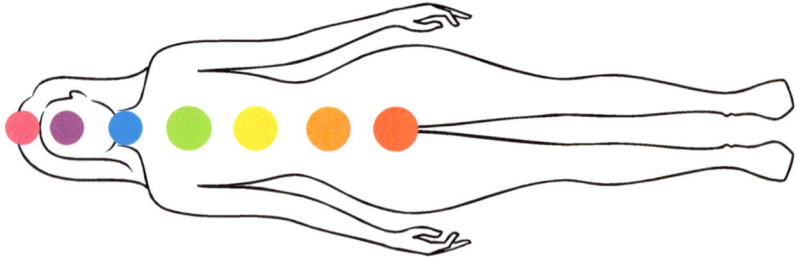

Chakra	Endocrine Gland	Related Organs	Function	Common Dysfunction	Music Notes
7th Crown	Pineal	Upper brain & right eye	Connection to spirit, harmony, joy & circadian rhythms	Feelings of alienation, confusion, depression, disconnection	B
6th Brow	Pituitary	Left eye, ears, nose, sinuses & lower brain	Insight, wisdom, compassion & humour	Sinus headache & blurred vision	A
5th Throat	Thyroid	Bronchia, lungs & larynx	Clear expression & communication	Throat problems, bronchitis & voice	G
4th Heart	Thymus	Heart & circulatory system	Sense of wellbeing, compassion & giving & receiving love	Cardiovascular disease, immune system & unresolved grief	F
3rd Solar Plexus	Pancreas	Digestive system	Positive self-esteem & self-will	Addiction, digestive problems, diabetes & lack of trust	E
2nd Sacral	Gonads	Reproductive organs	Emotional balance, relationships & community	Fluid imbalance & co-dependence	D
1st Root	Adrenals	Bones, spinal column & kidneys	Survival & community	Problems with lower back or hips, fatigue & lack of purpose	C

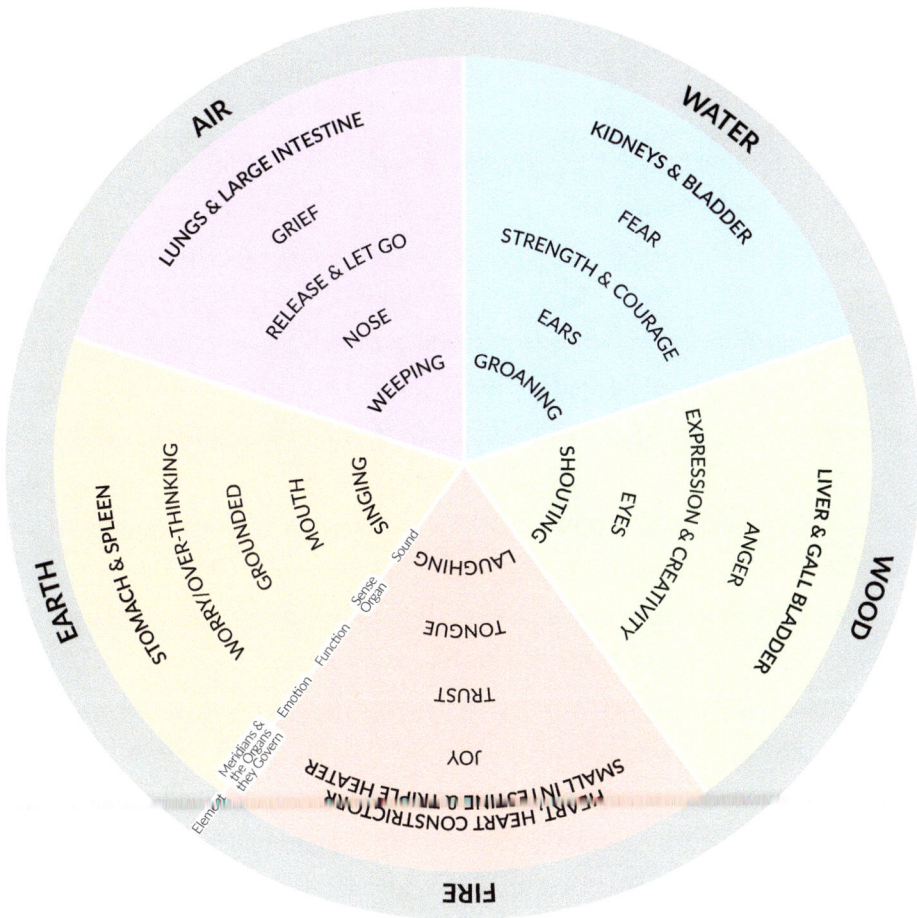

It is believed that chi travels through the network of meridian channels in synchronisation with the rhythm of nature. This is the biorhythm which is often called the biological clock. Any health problems with organs often arise at a particular time of day. Bilstrom (2024) in his article 'Morning Sunlight Strengthens Your Immune System by Optimizing Mitochondrial Function', explains that when we are exposed to the early morning sun (blue light) it sets our biorhythm and it also stimulates the process of creating new mitochondria cells.

It makes sense then that an increase in numbers of mitochondria improves energy production which of course supports the functioning of all of our organs and the systems they serve.

1–3 am	Liver	1–3 pm	Small Intestine
3–5 am	Lung	3–5pm	Bladder
5–7 am	Large Intestine	5–7 pm	Kidney
7–9 am	Stomach	7–9 pm	Heart Constrictor
9–11 am	Spleen/Pancreas	9–11 pm	Triple Heater
11–1 pm	Heart	11–1 am	Gall Bladder

In traditional Chinese medicine it is believed that we inherit an amount of energy from our parents called prenatal chi. Locke, in the book *Dancing the Elements: How to Dance Yourself to Physical and Spiritual Health with Wu Tao* explains that we deplete our chi/Qi reserves by over-work, stress, not enough sleep, deficient diet and too much sex or childbearing. Moderation is key to conserving our energy and protecting our storehouse of Qi.

The environment, our relationships, our emotions, thoughts, trauma and lifestyle choices influence our electromagnetic energy field/biofield. These can cause deficiencies, excesses, energy blockages, stagnations, the scattering of energy and distortions in the direction of flow of energy into our physical body, impacting our wellbeing. Self-care on all levels –physically, emotionally, mentally and spiritually can considerably help our general wellbeing, sense of vitality and rebalance our electromagnetic field, energy systems and energy flows.

All of this may sound complex, however there are some simple things that you can do to support your electromagnet field/biofield. You have already started doing this if you have tried the activities in Chapter One. Even the clearing space activity changes the environment and its energy flow within it. Creating a space that is practical, which contains the things that resonate and that are pleasing to you, will impact positively on your energy system and flow. There may be an internal clearing with the flow of tears through letting 'things' go. That's normal as you make way for the new, as well as you. A kind of feng shui.

The breathing and body scanning exercises reduce tension, bring relaxation, energy flow and energise at the same time. As the mind and the muscles of the body relax, the energy can flow to where it needs to go and deliver energy parcels efficiently.

It is my hope that going into some detail about how we operate as a 'perpetual human body' with three vital parts gives context and a foundation for discernment of your choices.

TASTER ACTIVITIES, TOOLS AND STRATEGIES

1. **Make a List with YOU on the Radar! (30 minutes)**
    - Make a list of all the activities that you spend time and energy on.
    - Then categorise your list into headings and place them in columns, with your name in the first column, e.g. Me ... Kids' Activities, Admin/ Finances, Chores, etc.
    - Ensure you have a list under your column. You could include items that you placed in the centre of your heart from your Personal Energy Tonic Treasury activity in Chapter One, or taster activities, tools and strategies for this chapter, etc.
    - Putting You at the first column gives you the visual permission for taking time to restore, while being able to see all the activities, responsibilities and commitments that you fulfil.
    - Put a colourful boundary in your favourite colour around your column to remind you that you are important, and that you matter.
    - You can use it as a tick-off list as well as it being a visual for your radar.
    - Add your self-care on the radar each week.

    Example:

...*Your Name*... I Forget You Not	Kids Activities	Admin	Chores	Appointments	Etc ...
_____	_____	_____	_____	_____	____
_____	_____	_____	_____	_____	____
_____	_____	_____	_____	_____	____

2. **Preparing for Schedules and Routines (1 hour)**

    If you don't have a diary and if cashflow allows, buy an A4 one that shows the full week over two pages. Or make a diary sheet for a full week.

3. **Non-Sleep Deep Relaxation (NSDR) (10 or 20 minutes)**

    NSDR was coined by Dr Andrew Huberman. This practice helps you get into a state of deep rest and relaxation without having a nap. It is deeply restorative to the mind while still being alert. This rest period can bring calm, focus and have you feeling energised. It can help you be more productive for the next bit of the day. It is also said to promote sleep – useful to recharge during the day and in the night if you are struggling to sleep.

    *   Visit YouTube – Andrew Huberman Non-Sleep Deep Rest (NSDR) to Restore Mental and Physical Energy to try a 10- or 20-minute NSDR.

4. **An Enjoyable Artistic Pursuit (30 minutes)**

    *   Carve out some time for yourself this week to creatively play.
    *   Continue with the same activity or choose another from your list of enjoyable artistic activities in Chapter One.

5. **Clearing Space: Room for You! (30 minutes)**

    Keep putting items in the box and aim to take them to the op shop by the end of the week.

6. **Journal Suggestions**

    *   Write down in your journal any thoughts or feelings about your findings so far, and anything that is happening for you in general.
    *   Which taster activities, tools and strategies worked well for you?
    *   Did anything stand out and how did you feel?
    *   Do you feel that any of the information, taster activities, tools and strategies will help reduce your fatigue signs?

- Have you noticed any changes in your fatigue signs, their severity and your energy levels?
- You may feel that you want to monitor your energy levels and fatigue signs. You can do this by regularly checking in with how you are feeling during certain activities and in different environments. There may even be a link with your energy levels/signs and certain places/activities.

7.   **My Personal Energy Tonic Treasury (20 minutes)**

In your journal draw your discerning resonant heart as shown below. It may need to take up the full page.

INNER HEART

- Write in the inner heart the points that have strongly stood out and resonated in the treasury of information, taster activities/ strategies/ tools that you want to include in your daily life **straight away**.
- Reflect on whether these things have been helpful towards reducing your fatigue signs and increasing your energy levels.
- Consult your journal and transfer anything else that is important to you. This may include the adapting or letting go of certain activities or routines, etc. that you have realised drain you of energy. It could also include ways that you can pace certain activities.

OUTER HEART

- Write in the outer heart the things you have identified that resonate with you and that you would like to change or include in your life **at some point in the future**.

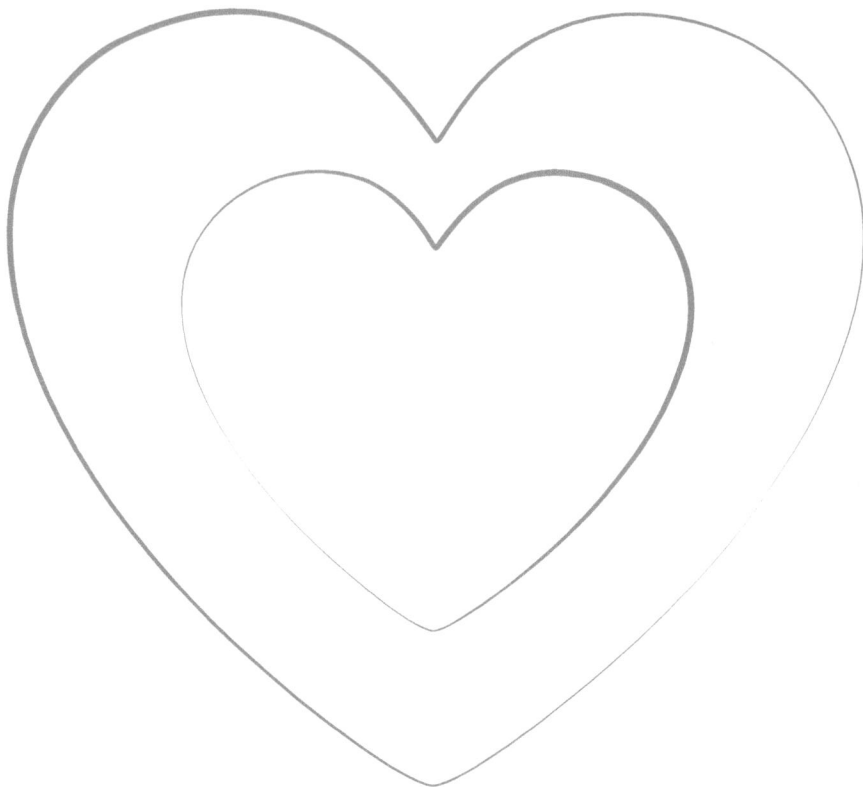

8. **Diarise (15 minutes)**

   - Put into your diary (or diary sheet) your entries from the inner heart of your Personal Energy Tonic Treasury from Chapter One and Chapter Two.

   - Keep the diary open and where it is visible. If you have a diary sheet, tack it on the wall where it will be hard to miss.

Congratulations! You have dedicated at least three hours and 15 minutes towards restoring your energy levels through these energy taster activities, tools and strategies. This doesn't include your journalling time.

References

1. Anderson, J.G., Anselme, L.C., Hart, K.H. (2017) *Foundations and Practice of Healing Touch,* p. 28–32.
2. Bilstrom, D. (15th May, 2024) *Morning Sunlight Strengthens Your Immune System by Optimizing Mitochondrial Function.* Available at: https://drdavidbilstrom.com/morning-sunlight-strengthens-your-immune-system-by-optimizing-mitochondrial-function/ (Accessed: September 2024).
3. Chang, S.T. (1986) *The Complete System of Self-Healing: Internal Exercises.*
4. Dorchester Health: The Benefits of Water. Available at: http://www.dorchesterhealth.org/water.htm (Accessed Jan 2014).
5. Geddes & Grosset (1999) *Practising Shiatsu.* Edition. Geddes & Grosset Ltd.
6. Gimbel, T. (2005) *The Healing Energies of Colour.* Gaia Books, p.61.
7. Karagulla, S. and Kunz, D. (1989) *The Chakras and the Human Energy Fields.* Wheaton, IL: Quest Books.
8. Locke, M. (n.d.) *Dancing the Elements: How to Dance Yourself to Physical and Spiritual Health with Wu Tao.* Book Pal, p 46.
9. Marieb, E. (1989) Chemistry Comes Alive, *Human Anatomy & Physiology.* Edition. Benjamin Cummings Publishing Co., Subs. Of Addison Wesley Longman, US, p.11.
10. *Metagenics for Life,* Metagenics Seminar (Oct–Nov 2009) *Energy for Life, natural approaches to the treatment of fatigue.*
11. Oschman, J. (2009) Charge transfer in the living matrix. *Journal of Bodywork and Movement Therapies,* 13, 215–220.

CHAPTER THREE

A Treasury of Energy Tonics

Breathing Well

As we discussed earlier, oxygen is important for the production process of ATP, the energy currency of the body.

From a traditional Chinese medicine perspective, the lungs control respiration; as Locke states the taking in of oxygen and pure Qi and the exhalation of carbon dioxide and toxins or impure Qi. The lungs are also responsible for the distribution of Qi through the body, sending it down from the lungs and dispersing it through the body. The lungs that receive oxygen/Qi have a special relationship with the skin and its protective functions, helping the skin to work as part of our immune system; the lungs circulate Qi to just under our skin.

It is with good reason then that we draw attention to how we breathe and how we can maximise oxygen intake. Some of the signs of fatigue that you identified in Chapter One will begin to reduce with regular attention to breathing and relaxation practice. Take note in your journal of any fatigue signs that are starting to dissipate and any rise in your energy levels.

✿ Just by taking ten minutes to notice and follow the pathway of your breath helps the body to relax (relaxation response), the body opens, our breathing becomes slower, fuller, and we naturally increase our capacity to take in more oxygen. This of course begins the restoration process and increase in energy levels.

☆ Harrison (2001) shares that when we relax completely, homeostasis (balance) is restored, which means the body is taking in just the right amount of oxygen it needs – not too much (which would stimulate the body) nor too little (which would starve it).

☆ When we slow everything down and take time out to notice the breath, we become more aware of our body, emotions and our thoughts. Being aware and listening in this way helps us know what our needs are. We can choose to be more responsive when we know what we need.

☆ The calming effect on the mind and the physical body makes the mitochondria happier and helps the production of our ATP energy currency.

☆ Attention to breathing reduces overthinking, clears the mind and brings clarity of thinking.

☆ Breathing with attention calms while energising.

☆ It's a form of resting the body and the mind.

☆ Breathing well supports sleep.

The Relaxation Response

Dr. Herbert Benson (2006) worked to build awareness of Mind Body Medicine, to validate it through research, and to bridge the gap between Western and Eastern medical practices. They found that meditation reduced metabolism, rate of breathing, heart rate, and brain activity. Dr Benson labelled these changes the 'relaxation response'. Through further study, Dr Benson found that the necessary two basic steps to elicit the relaxation response are: the repetition of a sound, word, phrase, prayer, or movement, and the passive setting aside of intruding thoughts and returning to the repetition. This can be done using any number of meditative techniques, such as diaphragmatic breathing, repetitive prayer, qigong, tai chi, yoga, progressive muscle relaxation, jogging, even knitting.

He explained that when high levels of stress hormones (cortisol) are secreted, often they can contribute to adrenal fatigue. The relaxation response is a helpful way to turn off the fight-or-flight response and bring the body back to pre-stress levels.

Hydration

Remember that every life-giving and healing process that happens inside of our body occurs in water, including the production of ATP. According to the European Food Safety Authority (EFSA) (2024), the recommended daily total water intake (from food and beverages) is:

2.0 l for women*
70–80% of daily water intake should come from drinks (water, beverages, etc.)
20–30% should come from food (fruits, vegetables, etc.)

Children:
2–3 years: 1,300 ml/day
4–8 years: 1,600 ml/day
9–13 years: 2,100 ml/day (boys) and 1,900 ml/day (girls)

Note that these recommendations are general guidelines and individual water needs may vary depending on factors such as climate, activity level and overall health.

The National Health Service (2024) in the UK lists the below signs of dehydration to include:
☘ Feeling thirsty
☘ Dark urine

---

*   Pregnant women: an additional 300 ml on top of the recommended 2 l daily intake.

- Not passing much urine
- Urine that smells
- Headaches
- Sunken eyes
- Lack of energy
- Feeling lightheaded
- Dry lips and skin
- Muscle cramps

Aerobic Exercise

Choosing a form of exercise that you enjoy is key to turning up. For me personally, putting the music on and having a good dance motivates me. Where there is motivation there is energy that carries you to the point of exercising. If it's swimming or walking, plan to do it.

- Exercise increases oxygen in circulation resulting in ATP production, increases metabolism and efficient use of energy.
- Increase in serotonin sees an increase in positive mood.
- Increases neurotransmitters (serotonin, dopamine, and norepinephrine) which brings calm, positive feelings, and energy.
- Sharpens cognition and memory because of more oxygen supplied to the brain.
- Release of physical and emotional symptoms related to stress making happy mitochondria producing energy.
- Increases stamina and strength.
- Boosts immune system and lowers inflammatory chemicals.
- Promotes sleep.
- Efficient healthier circulation system and respiratory systems which we need to deliver our oxygen.
- Can help clear blockages and free up energy in the bioenergy field related to stress and emotional blockages.

There was something interesting that I learned while reading the book *Ikigai: The Japanese Secret to a Long and Happy Life*, written by Garcia et al. (2017). The people who live the longest live in Japan. They don't do the most vigorous exercise but rather they move the most. One of the themes of the book is about the choices made in life being joyful ones, creating a flow in how they carry out their activities of daily living. This flow is synonymous with flowing energy. They keep busy in a relaxed flowing way as well as taking tea breaks, etc.

We could generally say that as solo mums we do a lot of moving. It is also explained in *Ikigai* that metabolism slows down 90% after 30 minutes of sitting. This lends itself to taking short rest breaks when life is super busy. The type of exercise described in *Ikigai* are the eastern disciplines for bringing body, mind and soul into balance like yoga, tai chi and qigong. Walking and dancing are also popular forms of exercise there.

It is still important to increase the heart rate, e.g. when walking to intentionally build up to a good brisk pace. Dancing certainly gets the heart rate and breath rate up too.

Stretching

- Stretching with good mindful breathing relaxes the muscles and mind. This makes space for energy flow.
- Increases blood flow to the muscles.
- Increases return of deoxygenated blood to the lungs exchanging for oxygen return.
- Increases oxygen supply to the muscles.
- Releases tension which frees up energy.
- Improves posture which again improves circulation by opening the body up.
- Can help sleep as with yoga.

Gentle Movement

- Tai chi is a low-impact, slow-motion exercise, breathing deeply and naturally. The movements are usually circular and gentle, the muscles are relaxed rather than tensed, the joints are not fully extended or bent, and the connective tissues are not stretched.
- The gentle movements unblock Qi so that it can flow through the body.
- Wu Tao is a form of dance therapy that is gentle and focuses on gentle movement to music. It stretches the meridian pairs that work together to promote the free flow of energy.
- There is a saying that gentle movement brings strength. There is also the idea that when we are gentle with ourselves mentally and emotionally, i.e. not being harsh with ourselves, there comes a strength and resilience.

Nutrition

- Consider energy input and output required, while thinking about the types of activities and work you do.
- Traditionally it has been recommended that we have a good-sized breakfast, medium-sized lunch and small dinner; however, have a read about the centenarian's diet after these bullet points. See what resonates with you.
- Spend longer chewing your meal. The extra breakdown of food really helps the absorption of energy-giving nutrients. It is said that the savouring of food, appreciation and enjoyment of it helps the breaking down and assimilation of the food further by our digestive system. This stimulates the further breaking down of food via saliva in the mouth and increases the intrinsic factor in the stomach. Intrinsic factor has an important role in the absorption of vitamin B12.

- Slowing down a bit at mealtimes helps us to sense when we are starting to get full and can prevent overeating. The energy that it takes to digest food is significant and therefore overeating can in fact make us feel sluggish, with less energy being used efficiently.
- Fresh food with a range of colours (different wavelengths of energy in the electromagnetic spectrum rainbow) usually ensures that we are getting enough of the vitamins and minerals that we need. You don't have to have the full spectrum of colour on one plate, but you can be mindful of the colours eaten throughout the day and where perhaps there may be a gap of colour in your diet.
- Most people that I have spoken to who suffer with fatigue and drink alcohol realise that it contributes to a reduction in their energy levels. Be mindful of how much alcohol is in the mix of your lifestyle.
- Slow-release carbohydrates such as oats ensure good energy supplies released during the day.
- Eating before 6 pm helps sleeping as the food is mainly digested by the time you go to bed. The energy can then go towards restoring us at a cellular level rather than the job of trying to digest a full tummy while trying to sleep.
- Weaver (2015) explains that it's important to understand the mechanisms of detoxification and elimination that your body utilises, because when they are compromised, typically energy is as well. She explains that numerous organs and body systems are involved in detoxification. They include: the liver, the colon, the kidneys, the skin and the respiratory system. Detoxification is a process that goes on inside of us all day, every day. The choices we make influence how efficiently the liver is able to do its job, and this significantly contributes to how we feel. She talks about 'liver loaders' as being alcohol, trans fats, refined sugars and caffeine. I also refer to the point that mitochondrial function is affected by toxicity resulting in a reduction in energy production. You may feel professional advice on a detox programme could be useful.

According to the World Health Organization, Japan has the highest life expectancy. Garcia et al. (2017) explain that it has the highest ratio of centenarians in the world. In Japan's province of Okinawa, life expectancy exceeds the national average. It is also the province that has managed to follow the Japanese Government's recommendations of eating less than ten grams of salt a day. The Okinawa diet is so often discussed around the world at panels on nutrition. The most concrete and widely cited data on diet in Okinawa comes from studies by Makoto Suzuki, a cardiologist at the University of the Ryukyus, who has published more than 700 scientific articles on nutrition and ageing in Okinawa since 1970. Bradley J. Willcox and D. Craig Willcox joined Makoto Suzuki's research team and published a book considered to be the bible on the subject, *The Okinawa Program*. As stated in *Ikigai*, the program reached the following conclusions:

- Locals eat a wide variety of foods, especially vegetables. Variety seems to be key … They ate an average of 18 different foods each day, a striking difference to the nutritional poverty of our fast-food culture.
- They eat at least five servings of fruits and vegetables every day. At least seven types of fruits and vegetables are consumed by Okinawans daily. The easiest way to check if there is enough variety is to ensure you are eating the rainbow … vegetables, potatoes, legumes and soy products such as tofu are the staples of an Okinawan's diet. More than 30% of their daily calories comes from vegetables.
- Grains are the foundation of their diet. Japanese people eat white rice every day, sometimes adding noodles. Rice is the primary food of Okinawa as well.
- They rarely eat sugar and if they do its sugar cane.

Garcia et al. also add that Okinawans eat fish an average of three times per week. There is also an 80% rule. When you notice that you are almost full but could have a little more, just stop eating. Food is served in small bowls or plates. One with rice, another with vegetables, a bowl of miso soup and something to snack on.

PQQ Connection with Biogenesis of Mitochondria

Biogenesis of the mitochondria is the self-renewal of mitochondria. New mitochondria are generated from the ones already existing.

Masahiko Nakano et al. (2012) researched the effects of an organic molecule pyrroloquinoline quinone (PQQ) on stress, fatigue and sleep. The results of the subjective evaluations were improved sleep, leading to reduced negative states, relief of fatigue and a rise in positive mood.

Kumazawa (1995) and his colleagues tested a range of foods for their PQQ levels. The highest levels were shown to be present in broad beans, parsley, green peppers, spinach, kiwifruit, green tea and oolong tea.

PQQ is also found in lower levels in celery, carrots, tofu, miso, potato, cabbage, sweet potato, banana, tomato, egg yolk and orange.

Whilst I am not an expert on supplements, it is also worth reading about the role of Coenzyme Q10 (ubiquinone) and magnesium in their roles within energy production. If you feel that supplements may have a larger role to play for you, consider speaking to a herbalist. It is well documented that increased magnesium levels are related to improved mitochondrial performance which affects ATP production. Magnesium can also help lower cortisol the stress hormone which can hamper ATP production.

Harmonising Energies and Flavours

Williams (1990) highlights that a healthy diet reflects all five flavours. This ensures that Qi and blood flows smoothly according to traditional Chinese medicine. Overemphasis on one flavour leads to disharmony of energy.

- Hot and spicy over-consumption impairs Qi and consumes bodily fluids.
- Balance sweet, sour, salty and bitter.
- Too much raw and cold food damages the energy of the spleen and stomach, leading to problems with digestive processes.

I hope this section has given you some food for thought. If you have special dietary requirements, it's always best to seek nutritional advice from a specialist/nutritionist.

TASTER ACTIVITIES, TOOLS AND STRATEGIES

1. **Herbert Benson's Relaxation Response (20–25 minutes) x2**
    1) Sit quietly in a comfortable position.
    2) Close your eyes.
    3) Deeply relax all your muscles, beginning at your feet and progressing up to your face. Keep them relaxed.
    4) Breathe through your nose. Become aware of your breathing.
    5) As you breathe out, say the word, "one", silently to yourself. For example, breathe in ... out, "one", in ... out, "one", etc. Breathe easily and naturally.
    6) Continue for 10 to 20 minutes.

    You may open your eyes to check the time, but do not use an alarm. When you finish, sit quietly for several minutes, first with your eyes closed and later with your eyes opened. Wait a few minutes before standing up.

    Do not worry about whether you are successful in achieving a deep level of relaxation. Maintain a passive attitude and permit relaxation to occur at its own pace. When distracting thoughts occur, try to ignore them by not dwelling on them and return to repeating "one".

    With practice, the response should come with little effort.
    Practise the technique **once or twice daily, but not within two hours after any meal**, since the digestive processes seem to interfere with the elicitation of the Relaxation Response.

    http://relaxationresponse.org/steps/

2. **Water Intake (10 minutes)**
   - Take note in your journal of what your daily water intake is. This means plain water intake. Then make a note of your beverage intake. Does not include alcohol.
   - Compare with the recommended intakes within this chapter.
   - Make a mental note of any changes to factor into your habits.

3. **Tea Break and The Art of Tea Drinking Meditation (20 minutes) x14**
   We usually have a chance to stop at some point in the day to make a brew and try to relax and hydrate. Tea is our time for downing the tools, STOPPING and hydrating. A way of pacing the day while taking in nutrients.
   - This week take stock of how often you sit down for a cup of tea and be intentional of having at least two tea breaks a day for 20 minutes each.
   - Have at least one of your cuppas in a quiet space where you can do the meditation that will be described shortly.
   - If you are doing a food shop this week and money allows ... treat yourself to a box of tea. Fruity tea, green tea, whatever you are drawn to. Otherwise, if you just love gumboot tea, go with it. Something that you like is the important part.
   - The time spent during the tea meditation has a luxuriousness and pampering aspect to it. The aim is that what might seem a quick tea break is going to be a sensory delight.
   - This is a practice of self-care that says you are worthy of enjoying your tea in the space and time that you have carved out for yourself. This self-care practice says you are important and essential! You matter.
   - This activity doesn't involve phones, reading magazines, books, listening to radios or watching the TV. There is just you and your tea.
   1) Sit down comfortably at the dining table with both feet flat on the floor. Your cup of tea is sitting on the table.

2) Make a loud sigh.

3) As you notice the steam rising from your cup you become aware of your feet resting on the floor, your body being supported by the chair, and of the natural rate of your breathing.

4) You think ... I am really going to enjoy and savour this tea and it's going to restore me with energy, hydration and nourishment.

5) You pick up your cup with both hands and feel the warmth of it in your hands.

6) You bring your cup towards your nose, close your eyes and inhale the tea's aroma. Take in the aroma and savour it.

7) Take a deep breath in and out and then place your lips on the cup. Gently sip your tea slowly. Notice the warmth, flavour and how the tea feels in your mouth. Gently swirl your tongue in the tea in your mouth.

8) Swallow your tea following its warmth in your throat, then your chest and down into your stomach.

9) Enjoy the feeling of radiating warmth, nurture and nourishment.

10) You feel a letting go of tension and relaxation while recharging.

11) Relax into the warm nurturing feeling and the pleasurable sensations. Let thoughts pass like clouds. Focus on your senses and the enjoyment of your tea.

12) Repeat with each sip the savouring through your senses.

13) You know you deserve and are worthy of the restoring break to relax and recharge.

14) When you have finished your tea notice how you feel in this moment physically, emotionally, mentally and the effect on your spirit.

15) Notice the level of relaxation that you are feeling and what your energy levels are compared to before enjoying your tea.

16) On a scale of 1–10 rate your energy levels. Low scores being low energy and high scores being higher energy levels.

17) Move forwards to the next part of your day.

4.   **Exercise (10 minutes)**

- Take note in your journal what kind of exercise you take and whether you feel you are taking enough of it.
- Ask if it is the right kind of exercise.
- What type of exercise do you enjoy? Could this be integrated into your day or week?

5.   **Nutrition (15 minutes)**

- Consider anything from your reading in this chapter that you want to change in terms of meals/foods.
- Are there any gaps in nutrition? What resonates regarding any initial changes that you might want to make?
- Add anything new on your food shop list for what the budget will allow.
- You may swap out some items which are not energy giving so that you can afford other items which are.
- Start with adding one or two food items to your shopping list each week.
- Consider if there is an item of food that you and the kids could grow in the garden at some point. It doesn't have to be initiated now, but it can be done at the right time in the future.

6.   **An Enjoyable Artistic Pursuit (30 minutes or more)**

- Carve out some time for yourself this week to creatively play.
- Continue with the same activity or choose another from your list of enjoyable artistic activities in Chapter One.
- Notice the level of relaxation that you are feeling and what your energy levels are compared to before.
- On a scale of 1–10 rate your energy levels. Low scores being low energy and high scores being higher energy levels.

7. ## Journal Suggestions
    - Write down in your journal any thoughts or feelings about your findings so far, and anything that is happening for you in general.
    - Which taster activities, tools and strategies worked well for you?
    - Did anything stand out and how did you feel?
    - Do you feel that any of the information, taster activities, tools and strategies will help reduce your fatigue signs?
    - Have you noticed any changes in your fatigue signs, their severity and your energy levels?
    - You may feel that you want to monitor your energy levels and fatigue signs. You can do this by regularly checking in with how you are feeling during certain activities and in different environments. There may even be a link with your energy levels/signs and certain places/activities.

8. ## My Personal Energy Tonic Treasury (20 minutes)
    In your journal draw your discerning resonant heart as shown below. It may need to take up the full page.
    ### INNER HEART
    - Write in the inner heart the points that have strongly stood out and resonated in the treasury of information, taster activities/ strategies/ tools that you want to include in your daily life **straight away**.
    - Reflect on whether these things have been helpful towards reducing your fatigue signs and increasing your energy levels.
    - Consult your journal and transfer anything else that is important to you. This may include the adapting or letting go of certain activities or routines, etc. that you have realised drain you of energy. It could also include ways that you can pace certain activities.
    ### OUTER HEART
    - Write in the outer heart the things you have identified that resonate with you and that you would like to change or include in your life **at some point in the future**.

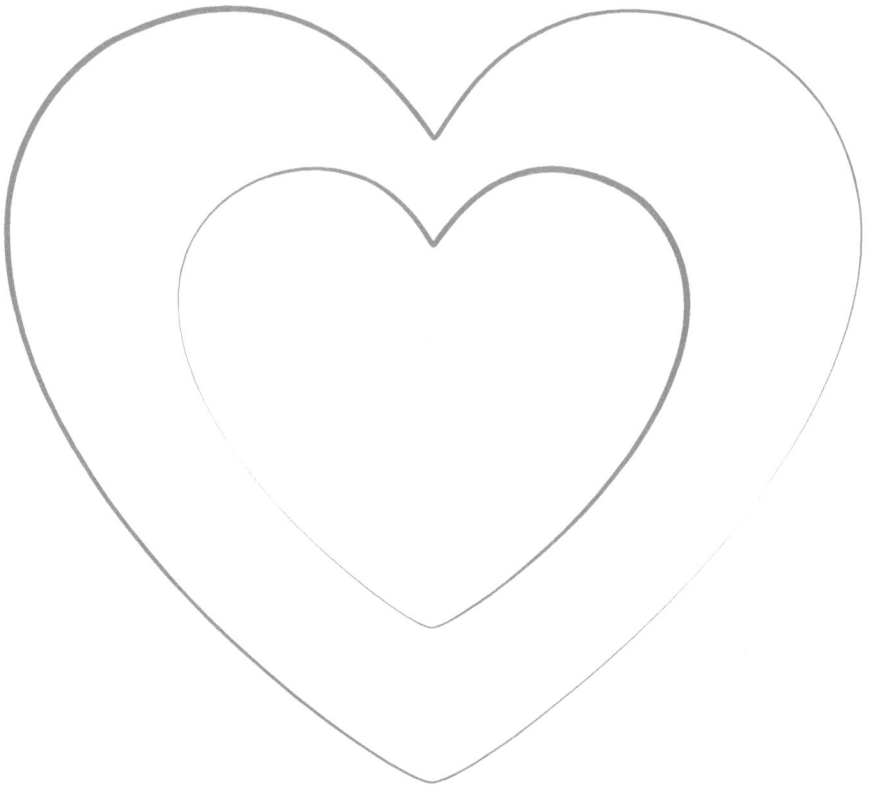

9.   **Diarise (15 minutes)**

   •   Put into your diary (or diary sheet) your entries from the inner heart
        of your Personal Energy Tonic Treasury activity from Chapter Three.

   •   Keep the diary open and where it is visible. If you have a diary sheet,
        tack it on the wall where it will be hard to miss.

   •   As you proceed through the week start adding energy scores at the
        start of the day, the end of the day, beside each activity and after
        each rest break. Use a score from 1–10. Lowest score as having
        low energy and highest scores more energy.

   •   The placing of your scores beside each activity will give you feedback
        about what really helps restore you and the activities that take most
        of your energy.

- Start to think about why some activities give low energy scores. Remember as human beings we function physically, emotionally and mentally which impacts the spirit. Does the activity or environment require intense focus and concentration? Or is it a very physically or emotionally demanding activity?
- If overall your energy scores are improving, then consider what you think is contributing to the increase in energy levels.
- Look at your scores after self-care activities, e.g. have your scores increased after a breathing strategy was used, or after a tea meditation, exercise, etc.? Be aware of what is working and building your energy reserves.

Congratulations! You have dedicated at least six hours and 50 minutes towards restoring your energy levels through these energy taster activities. This doesn't include your journalling time.

References

1. Benson, H. *The Relaxation Response*. Available at: *https://bensonhenryinstitute.org/mission-history/* (Accessed: August 2024).
2. Benson, H. (2006) Herbert Benson's *Steps to Elicit the Relaxation Response*. Available at: http://relaxationresponse.org/steps/ (Accessed: September 2024).
3. European Food Safety Authority. *Scientific Opinion on Dietary Reference Values for Water*. Available at: https://www.efsa.europa.eu/en/efsajournal/pub/1459 (Accessed: September 2024).
4. Garcia, H., Miralles, F. (2017) *Ikigai: The Japanese Secret to a Long and Happy Life*. Pub 2017 Penguin Random House UK, p. 123–128.
5. Harrison, E. (2001) *Meditation and Health*, Perth Meditation Centre, p. 63.
6. Kumazawa, T., Sato, K., Seno, H., Ishii, A., Suzuki, O. (1995) Levels of Pyrroloquinoline Quinone in Various Foods, *Biochemical Journal* April 1995; 307 (Pt2) 331–333.
7. Locke, M. (n.d.) *Dancing the Elements: How to Dance Yourself to Physical and Spiritual Health with Wu Tao*. Book Pal, p. 45–46.
8. Nakano, M., Yamamoto, T., Okamura, H., Tsuda, A., Kowatari, Y. (2012) Effect of Oral Supplementation with Pyrroloquinoline Quinone on Stress, Fatigue and Sleep, *Functional Foods in Health and Disease* 2012, 2(8): 307–324.
9. NHS. *Dehydration*. Available at: https://www.nhs.uk/conditions/dehydration/ (Accessed: September 2024).

10. Weaver. L. (2015) *Exhausted to Energised.* Pub 2015 Little Green Frog Publishing.
11. Willcox, B.J., Willcox, D.C., Suzuki, M. *The Okinawa Program: How the World's Longest-Lived People Achieve Everlasting Health – and How You Can Too.* Available at: http://www.penguinrandomhouse.com/books/190921/the -Okinawa-program-by bradley-j-willcox-md-d-craig-willcox-phd-makoto-suzuki-md-foreword-by-andrew-weil-md/ (Accessed: September 2024).
12. Williams, T. PhD. (1990) *Complete Chinese Medicine: A Comprehensive System for Health and Fitness.* Edition. Paragon Plus. p. 220–221.

CHAPTER FOUR

A Treasury of The Big Four:
Rest, Sleep, Play and Work

"Rest, sleep, play and work are termed as the 'big four' factors
a person should balance for the maintenance of health."
(Meyer 1977)

Rest: Restore and Restore

During my time working in neurological rehabilitation as an occupational therapist, we would recommend complete rest for patients. With our brain injury patients, we recommended regular rest periods as part of rehabilitation programmes. We termed the type of fatigue experienced by brain injury patients as neurogenic fatigue. Resting in this setting meant minimising sensory stimulation to the brain/nervous system as much as possible. Regular pacing with rest enhanced the healing process, maximising progress in rehabilitation. It meant the creating of boundaries and explaining to visiting friends and family that rest was part of recovering and a vital part of the rehabilitation process. Often people view rehab as full-on physical rehab. This is not so. There is a balance to be gained through activity and rest. Both are important. Sensory stimulation through the eyes, ears, skin, thoughts and emotions takes energy to process. Prior to head injury, many people equated rest and relaxation to mean listening to the radio, watching TV, reading, etc. In a way it is, but may have been categorised as being rest when in fact it can be classed as leisure or work. In the approach to fatigue management in this setting, everything that required attention and a response was classed as an activity.

While the chances are you may not have suffered a brain injury, it is valuable to be aware of this new meaning of resting. Sometimes it is apt just to switch off, be quiet without any stimulation at all to maximise recharging. If so tired that processing the words of a meditation is not possible, this is useful. I know it can be difficult to find this quiet time if you have younger children, but you may be able to pick your moments. It can be very valuable as a restorative strategy, particularly if you are having difficulties with concentration. If you can manage five or ten minutes of quiet time in a warm space, closing the curtains, closing your eyes and focusing on the pathway of your breath to clear the mind of other stimulating thoughts can help a lot.

Being responsive to how you are feeling is being responsive to those signposts that are telling you that you have overdone it and that you need to rest. Ideally, we hope to notice the signs much earlier, so that we can rest long before fatigue sets in. I understand the internal voice that says you can't rest – you can't relax because you have so much on your to-do list. Well, here's the thing – when you push forward, ignoring the signs, you are accumulating fatigue. There will be a time when you just *must* stop because you can't function any more. We want to avoid having to take days and weeks off because of fatigue. Planned breaks are far more enjoyable!

Ideally, we as busy women need to have planned rest periods during the day even if our energy levels are high. We need consistency as part of our daily routine rather than being dependent on the fatigue signs to tell us what to do. The point is to prevent the cycle of fatigue in the first place. Self-compassion to treat ourselves well so we have an energy supply in reserve.

It is important here to acknowledge our traits. We all have certain traits that don't always help our cause. Some people feel that they can't rest until all the jobs are done, then they feel they can give themselves permission to relax. How severe is this trait of soldiering on? Do all the jobs really get done? Will there always be something that needs to be done? How far does this extend before rest is deemed acceptable?

Then there is the perfectionist where there is resistance to resting until things are completed to a very high standard. An activity or job can't be left midway until it is done to the required high standards. Compromises feel difficult. Good or very good is not good enough. As solo mums, sometimes we feel that we need to make up for the shortfall of not having the support of a partner. We can try even harder and to be the best that we can be. This is totally understandable. The reality is that taking regular slots to restore is the answer to being the best that we can be. This will increase our energy to be productive and we will do it in a happier frame of mind. We most probably will flow through it nicely with ease. Gentleness with self is paramount.

Then there is the boom-and-bust type of behaviour. When we are feeling restored with our energy levels high, we go for it hell for leather, because we feel we can. No rest breaks, no restoring strategies or tools are used. The upshot of this is that we end up back at square one. The idea is having some form of pacing and balance that restores us of energy to enable us to give out energy.

Visualise a glass of water that keeps on pouring until it is empty – there is nothing more to give as it's all poured out. Then replace that visual with what tops up the glass for you and top it up frequently to maintain at least two-thirds of a glass full or more.

Although I have talked about complete rest, the strategies of breathing techniques and tea meditation are restful and recharging. It is for you to discern which strategy to use at a given time, by being in tune with how your energy levels are and what works best for you.

Consider asking for help from friends and family as an option. Asking for help can be scary. Some have a fear of people thinking that they might be struggling. Your phrasing when asking will help you with that. You can show that you are in control and are self-caring. "I would like some recharge time – could I drop the kids off for an hour?" Stick to the hour or the time frame that you have agreed to. I understand that it takes courage to ask. Consider who you feel you could ask and trust with your kids.

Think about giving your kids quiet wind-down time reading in their rooms in the evening, enabling you some rest time.

Sleep

According to Arden (2010), good-quality sleep recharges the batteries, facilitates regeneration of the cells and protein synthesis. It refreshes and energises and promotes myelin formation around the nerves which helps efficient firing of neurons. It supports concentration, new learning and memory.

The Stages of Sleep:
1. Transition: between waking and sleeping.
2. Light sleep (theta brainwaves): insomnia increases in periods of stress.
3. Deep sleep (slow delta waves): deep sleep boosts immune system. Sleep deprivation equals a suppressed immune system, and the body will ache.
4. REM (Rapid Eye Movement): if awakened people report vivid dreams. Metabolism goes up and energising neurotransmitters are active. REM should be 25% of the sleep time in healthy adults.

Atkinson (1989) states that if we are to restore our normal reservoir of energy, we need the right kind and right amount of sleep. A disturbance that keeps us awake too long, wakes us too early, makes us sleep too much, alters our normal cycle, or affects our sleep stages will affect our energy balance. When we are deprived of sleep for prolonged periods of time, we start to experience increased fatigue, irritability and difficulties with concentration. If we do not rest, the symptoms progress to deterioration of motor function, decreased motivation and even hallucination.

The sleep cycle/circadian rhythm is affected by daylight and darkness.
- The light and dark are received by the retina of the eye.
- The pineal gland responds to the light and suppresses melatonin telling the brain that it is daytime and helps us to wake up in the morning.
- The pineal gland responds to the dark and produces melatonin which induces sedation/sleep.

To set the circadian rhythm to match the natural day/night cycle, ensure some exposure to daylight. There is growing literature now that talks about the overuse of sunglasses limiting the receiving of natural light affecting our circadian rhythms.

Promoting Quality Sleep:
- Have exposure to natural daylight to set your circadian rhythm for the day/night cycle.
- Aim to rise at the same time each day and go to bed at the same time. This can be challenging with babies and very young children, I know!
- Rest or relax during the day rather than taking a nap. If you need a nap, ensure it is before 3 pm and set a timer. Mums with young babies or toddlers often take the opportunity to recharge with a nap when their babies nap.
- Have a balance of activity/exercise with some rest during the day.
- No caffeine after lunch, avoid eating after 6 pm, have a lighter evening meal and avoid alcohol 4–6 hours before going to bed.
- Reduce or omit alcohol, eat a fresh, balanced diet, receive support to quit smoking if you smoke.
- If you have a television, phone and/or computer in your bedroom, remove them if possible. This ensures there is no disturbance from EMFs and notifications. The bedroom should be associated with sleep. If you must have your phone in your room, put it on flight mode.
- Avoid looking at television, computers and phone screens two hours before going to bed. Dim the lighting so that the circadian rhythm can move through its cycle. If your retina is exposed to light, it will trick your pineal gland into thinking it is morning and time to wake up.
- Improve air quality (open bedroom window), reduce temperature but ensure that you are warm enough.
- Use blackout curtains, particularly if there are bright streetlights that disturb your sleep.
- Consider the comfort of your bed and pillows.

❀ If you can't switch off your mind because you worry you might forget something for the next day, put the items on your mind on your list/diary and then relax.

❀ If you have a lot on your mind, you could write in your journal and pour all your concerns onto the page. Then let it go and relax.

❀ Taking a bath or shower two hours before sleep raises and then reduces body temperature which is conducive to sleep.

❀ Relax the senses before bed. Avoid stimulating thriller movies or any screen time two hours before sleep.

❀ Try relaxing music, lavender essential oil, gentle stretching, a glass of warm milk.

❀ Jamie Clements' *The Breath Space* on YouTube does a great guided breathing routine to prepare for sleep right before you want to go to sleep. (Remember to remove your device after or turn onto flight mode). Simply paying attention to your breathing in and out of your nose to induce relaxation for sleep is also useful.

❀ If you can't sleep after 20 minutes, get up and do something like listen to calm music, or make a hot drink if you haven't already before bed.

❀ Be patient as it can take a while to work out a sleep routine that suits you.

Play

Under the topic of play I want to touch on the benefits of hobbies, leisure, laughter, humour, the benefits of play and play personalities.

When we invest time and energy in our interests, hobbies, and leisure pursuits we create energy flow that is restorative, reduces tension and lifts the spirits.

A literature review done by Suto (1998) on approaches to leisure in occupational therapy concluded that although leisure had been identified by many authors as an important aspect of a balanced lifestyle, it was afforded less status than work.

I must agree that when the stress kicks in and life becomes busy, play-time/leisure/hobbies appear to be the first things that get the heave-ho. Even though we know at a conscious level that these activities would be a great stress reliever, they still seem to drop off the side of a cliff. We get that voice that says it's not a priority, I don't have time for this, my list is too long, too much to do and everything will fall apart if I dare to play and relax. What good is my impassioned hobby going to be when I need to work extra hours to pay the bills? I am running out of time to make that costume for Amy for the school show. Well, taking time out to do your impassioned hobby helps creativity and efficiency because you are firing on all cylinders.

Prioritising and engaging in a hobby is also a great means of experiencing joy. Joy, as in the lifting of our spirits, is essential for our wellbeing and we choose hobbies and interests to help us do this. Hobbies are classed as leisure and recreational activities. I liked the definition of recreation by *Merriam-Webster* (2024) on their online dictionary as being the refreshment of strength and spirit after work. They define a hobby as a pursuit outside one's regular occupation engaged in especially for relaxation. The *Cambridge Dictionary* (2024) defines leisure as activities people do when they are not working to relax and enjoy themselves. **Where there is an interest in enjoyment, meaning and purpose, there is also motivation. Where there is motivation there is energy.** Such is the great importance of joy and enjoyment that I have dedicated the following chapter to this subject.

Fun and laughter is also worth noting here too. What if we make conscious space and time to say to ourselves, right, it's just time to have a laugh? Put on a great comedy sketch or catch up with bubbly friends. (I'm not necessarily talking champagne here!) I read a great article in the UK publication of *Occupational Therapy News* written by Hortop (2008) about a therapist who used laughter and humour where appropriate in her approach with her patients. It was explained that the mere anticipation of laughter decreases the anxiety response of cortical production. The smiling releases feel-good endorphins that have the same effect on our bodies as morphine, which reduces pain perception, inflammation and relaxes us. Laughter therapy is the active pursuit of happiness through humour, positivity, enjoyment and feeling good.

There is various research out there to support that humour and having fun boosts our biochemistry and immune system. Laughing brings a light-heartedness, an air of taking things less seriously and it helps us to release tension. It is also known to improve cognitive function, and laughter provides a form of exercise as well as relaxation. I certainly feel energised after a good laugh while simultaneously feeling that I have well and truly let go.

When it comes down to the nitty gritty, all the things that we associate with hobbies, leisure, fun, laughter, humour and play reduce stress, stimulate the brain and improve its function, increase emotional wellbeing, boost productivity and in effect prevent burnout and restore us.

According to Play Australia (2024), play is not just essential for kids; it can be an important source of relaxation and stimulation for adults as well. In our hectic, modern lives, many of us focus so heavily on work and family commitments that we never seem to have time for pure fun. Somewhere between childhood and adulthood, we've stopped playing … Adult playtime is a time to forget about work and commitments. The focus of play is on the actual experience, not on accomplishing any goal.

Play can include the following benefits:

- Relieve stress. Play is fun and can trigger the release of endorphins, the body's natural feel-good chemicals. Endorphins promote an overall sense of wellbeing and can even temporarily relieve pain.
- Improve brain function. Playing chess, completing puzzles, or pursuing other fun activities that challenge the brain can help prevent memory problems and improve brain function. The social interaction of playing with family and friends can also help ward off stress and depression.
- Stimulate the mind and boost creativity. Young children often learn best when they are playing – and that principle applies to adults as well. You'll learn a new task better when it's fun and you're in a relaxed and playful mood. Play can also stimulate your imagination, helping you adapt and problem solve.
- Improve relationships and your connection to others. Sharing laughter and fun can foster empathy, compassion, trust and intimacy with others.

Play doesn't have to be a specific activity; it can also be a state of mind. Developing a playful nature can help you loosen up in stressful situations, break the ice with strangers, make new friends, and form new business relationships.

Keep you feeling young and energetic. In the words of George Bernard Shaw, 'We don't stop playing because we grow old; we grow old because we stop playing.' Playing can boost your energy and vitality and even improve your resistance to disease, helping you feel your best.

https://www.playaustralia.org.au

Dr Stuart Brown founded the National Institute for Play and is dedicated to advancing society's understanding and application of play. Brown states that the drive to play is as fundamental as our drives for food and sleep. On the National Institute for Play website Dr Stuart Brown's play personalities can be found. Eight play personalities were discerned from thousands of interviews and observations. Most people tend to have one dominant play personality type and one or two minor ones. The play personalities model has helped adults who have 'lost' their play life to identify and rekindle it. It is Dr Brown's observation that actualising one's deepest talents is associated with an engaged sense of play. Keeping play in one's life is vital to a successful life journey. Adults who do not regularly activate their play nature may experience their lives as tinged with depression and may lack optimism, adaptability and resilience to perform well in their work and family life.

The Eight Play Personalities:

1. The Collector: the collector of objects or experiences and can be solitary or with social connections (coins, wine, shoes, videos, etc).
2. The Competitor: competitive games with specific rules (video games, playing sport or watching sport).
3. The Creator/Artist: joy found in making things or making things work and mending things (painting, pottery, knitting, gardening, decorating a room).

4.   The Director: plays by planning, organising and executing scenes and events (film-makers, party planners, excursion planners).

5.   The Explorer: physically going to explore places/emotionally searches for a new feeling or a deepening of the familiar through music, movement. Or researching out a new subject.

6.   The Joker: practical jokes and clowning around.

7.   The Kinesthetes: people who like to move and some need to move to think. This can include athletes and people who find themselves happiest moving as part of dance, swimming, walking, playing football. While kinesthetes may play sports, competition is not the main focus – it's a way of engaging in movement.

8.   The Storyteller: imagination is key to the joy of play. (Novelists, playwrights, cartoonists or screenwriters, or reading novels and watching movies. Performers are storytellers, through acting, dance, lectures or magic tricks).

https://nifplay.org/what-is-play/play-personalities/

From the research regarding play I think we can deduce that play is a very important form of self-care and to be guarded from falling off the cliff when life gets too busy or stressful. If play becomes less frequent, it's time to stop and review the busy schedule and reprioritise some things so that we can remain grounded in play and do what we enjoy.

Work

In Chapter One you will remember the Life Balance taster activity. You were asked to work out the number of hours that you spent in each life area of rest/sleep, self-care, leisure and productivity/work. There was the accompanying quote from Turner (2002) that activities are the means through which people control the balance in their lives … People make decisions about what they will and won't do and when, where how and with whom they will do it.

Turner's research showed that the optimal percentage of time allotted to each of the four categories of healthy individuals per day is as follows:

Rest/Sleep	=	33%	(8 hours)
Self-Care	=	11.2%	(2 hours 40 mins)
Leisure	=	9.2%	(4 hours 40 mins)
Productivity/Work	=	36%	(8 hours 40 mins)

When you compare the percentage of rest/sleep (33%) with productivity/work (36%) there is minimal difference, especially if you view the percentages in terms of restoring energy. It could be argued that the self-care percentage of 11.2% takes the energy-restoring or topping up to 44.2% which far outweighs the expenditure of energy of productivity/work.

When everything we do can be viewed as energy-restoring and energy expenditure, we see that our choices are consequential in maintaining the balance of our health and energy levels. I note that the leisure activities featured highly in these healthy individuals. While four hours and 40 mins a day of leisure may not be feasible for some, we can at least move it along in our priority list and aspire to an allotted time each day.

The at Work Australia (2024) website lists the health benefits of work. It talks about meaningful work being essential to wellbeing. Work that satisfies you and fulfils a purpose also helps you to create a sense of personal achievement, identity and purpose, learn a new skill and gain experience, progress your career, connect with people and your community, contribute to something and achieve success, improve mental health, build a routine and find work-life balance.

In Chapter Seven under the topic of ikigai I will focus more on work in terms of purpose and meaning.

It goes without saying that the type of work you do will affect how you take care of yourself in the workplace. Highly physical work may require you to have a sit-down break and a higher calorie lunch. Sedentary work might require you to have a short walk in your break and a lighter lunch. If you work in a noisy environment you might need to find a quieter space and so on. Be self-compassionate in listening and responding to what you require for your energy top-ups at work. Your type of work may also inform you of the kind of rest, leisure activities and routines that you choose outside of work.

TASTER ACTIVITIES, TOOLS AND STRATEGIES

I recommend that you take a few weeks with this chapter if you feel you need to. Three weeks is also good while you keep up the commitment and momentum flowing. Do not be put off by the number of activities. Have a playful approach to exploring and bringing together information in these activities that are categorised to support your energy levels. There is some contemplating for you about habits and routines, putting together your energising jigsaw puzzle.

1.   **Supportive Habits and Routines: Favourite Effective Breathing Exercises to Restore your Energy Levels (20 minutes)**
     - Review in your diary and reflect in your journal which breathing exercises have increased your energy levels, the ones you enjoy and the ones that may have dissipated some of your fatigue signs.
     - Choose your favourite breathing exercises and consider whether there could be set times of the day that you might use them, as well as using on an 'as and when needed' basis.
     - Write anything that you want to include from this section about new habits/routines and breathing exercises in your Personal Energy Tonic Treasury.

2.   **Supportive Habits and Routines: Rest Breaks to Restore Your Energy Levels (20 minutes)**
     - Write and reflect in your journal about whether you have set scheduled rest periods.
     - If not, consider how rest periods could become part of your routine.

Whether it be complete quiet, a breathing exercise, a tea meditation or something else. At least two 20-minute slots during the day would be fantastic.

- Write your findings in your Personal Energy Tonic Treasury.

3. **Supportive Habits and Routines: Mealtimes to Restore Your Energy Levels (20 minutes)**
   - Look at your habits and routines in terms of mealtimes. Can older kids help with aspects of meal prep, or even be rostered to take responsibility for making a full meal?
   - Consider the time of meals in relation to the sleep promotion points in this chapter.
   - Write anything that you might want to change in your mealtime habits/routines in your Personal Energy Tonic Treasury.

4. **Supportive Habits and Routines: Nutrition to Restore Your Energy Levels (20 minutes)**
   - Consider any new foods to put on the shopping list this week.
   - Reflect on the information in Chapter Three. Take note of any changes you may have made to your eating and nutritional habits, how your energy levels are and what is happening with your fatigue signs.
   - Write any significant items/changes in your Personal Energy Tonic Treasury.

5. **Supportive Habits and Routines: Sleep to Restore Your Energy Levels (30 minutes)**
   - Look at your existing routines and habits in terms of sleep and reflect on the information in this chapter.
   - Identify anything that resonates with you that you want to change to promote better sleep.
   - You could reflect on this for you and the family. Write anything that you may want to integrate in your Personal Energy Tonic Treasury.

6.   **Supporting Habits and Routines: Exercise to Restore Your Energy Levels (20 minutes)**

   - Consider from the last chapter any forms of exercise you may have identified that you enjoy, or anything new that you might like to try.
   - If you have anything to add to your routines/habits in terms of exercise, place it in your Personal Energy Tonic Treasury.

7.   **Supporting Habits and Routines: Playtime (Hobbies, etc.) to Restore Your Energy Levels (1 hour 30 minutes)**

   - Reflect on how much playtime you engage in and what play might look like for you.
   - Make a list in your journal of what you used to play as a kid. If you need a bit of help reminiscing, start with your earliest memory of playing, then 5–10 years of age, 11–15 years, 16–21 years and onwards to the present day.
   - Circle the most fun play activities.
   - Reflect in your journal about the play personalities and what resonates with you. Is your attention drawn to any play activities or styles that you want to rekindle? What styles/activities make your heart sing? What styles/activities make time disappear and make you feel in your flow?
   - Go to The National Institute for Play website https://nifplay.org/what-is-play/play-personalities/ and take the Play Personality Quiz and reflect in your journal.
   - Is there any play activity that you have thought you would like to do?
   - If anything resonates with you, transfer it into your Personal Energy Tonic Treasury.
   - This week have one playdate with yourself for at least 30 minutes as part of self-care and restoring your energy.
   - Rate your energy levels before and after your playtime activity as you have done with other activities.

8.   Supportive Habits and Routines: Asking for Help to Restore Your
Energy Levels (1 hour)
- Consider who you could ask for help in having the kids for a time
while you recharge your batteries.
- Make a list of who you could trust, how long you would need and
whether you could ask for a regular time slot each week or even
every fortnight.
- Asking for help can also open doors for you to go out on your own
to a leisure/hobby club or exercise group, etc.
- Once you feel happy with who you have chosen, think about what
you would do in that time. **Chores are strictly not allowed.** This
activity is about restoration and balance with self-care. This is the
time to draw a circle around you, the time and activity.
- When you are happy with your choices and what you plan to do with
the time, contact the person/people to ask about the possibility.

9.   An Enjoyable Artistic Activity (30 minutes or more)
- Carve out some time for yourself to creatively play.
- Continue with the same activity or choose another from your list
of enjoyable artistic activities list in Chapter One.
- Notice the level of relaxation that you are feeling and what your
energy levels are compared to before enjoying your artistic activity.
On a scale of 1–10 rate your energy levels. Low scores being low
energy and high scores being higher energy levels.
- Are there any of these enjoyable artistic pursuits that you would
like to carry on into your routines? If there is anything that stands
out enter it into your Personal Energy Tonic Treasury.

10.   Journal: Supportive Habits and Routines to Restore Your Energy
Levels (2 hours)
- Write down in your journal any thoughts or feelings about your
findings and anything that is happening for you in general physically,
emotionally, mentally and spiritually.

- Over the next two or three weeks start to play with all the information that you have gathered in your Personal Energy Tonic Treasury; experimenting on the pages of your journal with new routines/habits that you want to include to restore your energy levels.
- Make a table for the seven-day week and put in any work commitments.
- If journalling is useful to you make sure that a journalling slot is integrated.
- If you go to work, ensure you get your breaks and lunch. If you need a change in environment or quiet space, consider going for a walk or finding an empty office, etc.
- Place in your routines the activities that will make the biggest difference to your energy levels.
- Pace the day, particularly during intense activities.
- Take note of when you know you function at your best, e.g. early morning or afternoon and plan more demanding activities at those times followed with a rest break.
- You may find you want to prioritise some things that are non-negotiable in the knowledge that some activities significantly restore you.
- When you feel satisfied with what you have on paper, diarise it all and give it a trial. Make notes of any tweaks and changes that will make things run more smoothly. Treat this as experimental play.

11.   **Diarise: Supportive Habits and Routines to Restore Your Energy Levels (1 hour)**
- Add to your diary/diary sheet from the above task.
- As you proceed through the week start adding your energy levels at the start of the day, end of the day and beside each activity. Use a score from 1–10. Lowest score as having low energy and highest scores having more energy.

- The placing of your scores beside each activity will give you feedback about what really works in the big picture of your new habits and routines.
- The plan is that your energy becomes more easily topped up to higher levels consistently with your new habits and routines.
- Take note of the quality of your sleep and what your energy levels are like before sleeping and upon waking.

Congratulations! You have dedicated at least eight hours and 30 minutes towards restoring your energy levels through these energy taster activities. This doesn't include your personal journalling time.

References

1. Arden, J. B. (2010) *Rewire Your Brain: Think Your Way to a Better Life*. Wiley.
2. Atkinson, H. (1989) *Women and Fatigue*. Edition. Papermac.
3. atWork Australia. *Health benefits of work*. Available at: https://www.atworkaustralia.com.au/health-benefits-of-work/ (Accessed: September 2024).
4. Brown, S, *Play Personalities: What Are Your Play Personalities?* Available from: https://nifplay.org/what-is-play/play-personalities/ (Accessed September 2024).
5. Hortop, A. (2008) Laughter therapy: extended scope of practice or just part of the job? OTnews May 2008.
6. Meyer, A. (1977) The philosophy of Occupational therapy. *American Journal of Occupational Therapy*, 31(10), 639–42.
7. Play Australia, *The Benefits of Play for Adults: How Play Can Improve Your Health, Work, and Family Relationships*. Available at: https://www.playaustralia.org.au (Accessed September 2024).
8. Suto, M. (1998) Leisure in Occupational Therapy. *Canadian Journal of Occupational Therapy*, 65 (5), 271–78.
9. Turner, A., Foster, M.A. and Johnson, S.E. TDipCOT MA FCOT (2002). *Occupational Therapy and Physical Dysfunction: Principles, Skills and Practice*, 5e. 5th Edition. Churchill Livingston.

CHAPTER FIVE

A Treasury of Joy

The American Psychological Association defines joy as a feeling of extreme gladness, delight, or exultation of the spirit arising from a sense of wellbeing or satisfaction. The feeling of joy may take two forms: passive and active. Passive joy involves tranquillity and a feeling of contentment with things as they are. Active joy involves a desire to share one's feelings with others. It is associated with more engagement of the environment than passive joy. The distinction between passive and active joy may be related to the intensity of the emotion, with active joy representing the more intense form. Both forms of joy are associated with an increase in energy and feelings of confidence and self-esteem.

The Art and Science of Joy website is a lovely, uplifting read. They have a mission to inspire and empower you to find more joy in your life. They describe that the foundation for a joy-filled life is built on taking care of our own emotional, mental, physical and spiritual wellbeing. And as we humans are social animals, we also need a sense of genuine belonging to flourish. With a strong base of wellbeing and belonging, we have the strength to have a positive impact on others … through our thoughts, words and actions and thereby bring even more meaning and joy to our lives. They state that wellbeing, belonging, positive impact and fun are four simple and yet powerful ingredients to help you live a joy-filled life.

They provide the following framework guide for finding your joy:

Wellbeing	Belonging	Positive Impact	Fun
Physical	Family	On Other People	Entertainment
Emotional	Friends	On the Planet	Hobbies
Mental	Community		
Spiritual	Work/School		

Everyone has their own recipe for finding joy and we can experiment and play to find what makes us tick.

I would like to share two stories. They each relate to my mother and father and how enjoyable activities deeply affected their lives when they were unwell.

When I was in my forties, my mother was diagnosed with breast cancer. She went through recommended treatments of mastectomy, chemotherapy and radiation. Unfortunately, she received an incorrect dose of chemotherapy and fought for her life in intensive care. Mum described that she had a near-death experience. She was given a clear message that for her future health she needed to dance every day. Specifically, she was told that dancing was from now on her immunity. Interesting. She indeed loved to dance and was a member of her local dance school. After being discharged from hospital and when she had the strength, she got herself to dance class, and friends would take her when they could. The dance teacher placed a chair at the back of the studio as a place for her to rest when she needed to. The fatigue and nausea were sometimes severe. Pacing herself, dance became Mum's rehabilitation and the dance teacher her therapist. She danced her way to gently building back her strength and health. Mum declined further chemotherapy, and the joy of dance was a significant part of her medicine which has kept her fit and well.

This wholeness of integrating and flowing well physically, emotionally and mentally lifts the spirit. This is fundamental here. Mum was engaged pretty much daily in the art and enjoyment of dancing with her friends, and it became her personal medicine.

I have another story to share. My father had been admitted to a nursing home. He had been diagnosed with Parkinson's disease many years prior and

Mum looked after him for as long as she could. My daughter and I went back to the UK to visit family (the trip I spoke about earlier). When we went to see Dad, his condition had deteriorated to the point where he wasn't able to communicate or initiate movement and needed assistance with all aspects of care. It was the first time I had seen him in a while, and he was almost unrecognisable – he held a fixed grimace, like a frozen mask. We took him to the seafront in his wheelchair where a most magical experience occurred.

We stopped on the promenade to look at the sea and enjoy the fresh air together. My daughter loved to play football. She had brought her football with her, and gently started kicking it towards him. A light immediately came on for my dad. A facial expression with a smile broadening across his face. Literally a sparkle in his eyes, like his spirit was activated. He looked like the man I always knew. He then initiated sitting up straight in the wheelchair, he flexed at the hip, extended his knee and coordinated accurately kicking the ball. This happened consistently back and forth. It didn't stop there. He then turned to me and started talking. I was overcome with joy. We got to see him again.

There is a background story to this. Dad, from a very young age, spent most of his time with a football and playing football for various teams in Yorkshire. He was an excellent football player, and it was his life's blood. If he wasn't playing it, he would watch it on TV. Unfortunately, he sustained a knee injury which ended his career. He was understandably devastated that he could no longer play at that level anymore. We shared what had happened with the staff upon our return to the nursing home, and in turn, they could encourage movement and wellbeing by integrating football activities into his daily routine.

The energy of joy or enjoyment I believe brings a convergence of wholeness physically, emotionally, mentally and spiritually within our hearts. Joy and enjoyment appeared to activate Dad on all these levels when previously physical movement and speech couldn't be coordinated, muscles were stiff and he had no facial expression. All the difficulties melted away. His enjoyment and passion for football was the catalyst and spark of his innate ability to integrate physically, emotionally, mentally and spiritually to kick the ball. The sudden ability to initiate and control movement was not through thinking it into being. It came from his heart, the enlivening and motivating spark of his spirit in his enjoyment.

When Dad was still living at home, Mum had taken him to dance classes for Parkinson's sufferers. This also made a difference. Dance wasn't really his thing, but music absolutely was. The rhythm of the musical beats helped him to initiate movement and stepping in time consistently.

The true essence of occupational therapy when unconstrained by systems, is the use of meaningful and purposeful activities with patients in their rehabilitation goals. This encompasses the balance of physical, emotional, mental and spiritual aspects of being human in the approach to rehabilitation. It is a wonderful profession when able to be practised in the fullest to which it was intended. The truth is, we can all practise our own occupational therapy when it comes to our wellbeing and restoration. Engaging in joyful activities is a fantastic way to do this. Knowing what resonates with us physically, emotionally and mentally is key … this lifts the spirit.

I trained in a form of dance movement therapy which incorporates the foundations of traditional Chinese medicine (TCM). The heart in TCM has the function of housing the spirit which radiates outwards. When we live life in balance in accordance with who we truly are, the spirit rests in the heart joyfully. The heart constrictor functions as a protector of the heart and our spirit. The heart constrictor is also symbolic of healthy boundaries in order for needs to be met.

There are times when we review our priorities in terms of how we are living and ask whether our enjoyment needs are being met. Asking deep questions about what makes us tick and our hearts sing is important. There are times that we start to ask ourselves these kinds of questions when we lose ourselves. Midlife crisis springs to mind as one of these instances.

The word 'heart' holds the words 'hear' and 'art'. Can we hear our art through our heart? Listen to your heart and you will know your art? Can we ask who art you? What speaks to your heart? What speaks to your heart leads to your spirit and joy. The true you.

Amongst the stressors we need enjoyment more than ever before. Fear and worry are a killjoy. They also disrupt restoration, relaxation and drain us of energy. It's an absolute must for us to include activities of enjoyment in our lives. Joy is a guiding light. When it becomes a priority for us, we are winning the inner spiritual conflict that happens between fear, worry and joy. We feel better on all levels. I also notice that when I self-care with joyful activities, answers come to problems and concerns without thinking about them. When I think back to the many times when I was in anguish, overthinking and worrying about so many things, I wish I was guided to just lay it down for an hour or two and direct myself to a fun activity. I know now that this would have led me to asking the right questions and asking the right people instead of trying to figure things out on my own. In traditional Chinese medicine, overthinking and worrying interrupts our ability to cognitively work things out. Being grounded in joy in who we truly are and doing joyful things socially, tends to lead us to places and people who have similar hearts to ours. This can further add to our like-minded/-hearted support network. Asking ourselves who we truly are brings about growth and living true to ourselves.

My sister, who is also a solo mum, shared that there was a particular time when she was having it rough and dealing with so many issues when her son was very young. She said what helped was putting her son's favourite singing and dancing programme on. They would just jump and dance around the living room singing at the top of their voices. She felt, after letting go singing, dancing, laughing and having fun, that there was a sense of relief, and that the situation looked and felt less severe.

My daughter was a teenager when my husband and I separated, and she was starting to find her independence. After a while of getting sorted out (i.e. our living situation and returning to work in the health system), I started to let go a little and find enjoyable activities for me again. Fridays after work was relaxing and restoring night. My daughter would often go to her dads on Friday nights. I would come home from work, go buy a pizza, a bottle of red wine, relax in the living room, wine and dine myself, run a hot bath, and languish in it with music playing on my iPad, singing along to my favourite songs. I felt worth it, and I was enjoying myself!

After a while it became clear that working back in the healthcare system was not the right choice for me. I decided to hand in my notice and look to further build my business. I joined an affordable women's gym which had an array of classes including Zumba and spinning bike classes. I loved them! I made some new friends there and did feel a new sense of belonging. There was a sauna to relax in after if I had the time. Interestingly, my daughter also joined the same gym. I do feel that when we attend to ourselves then the kids also follow suit to do what they need to do.

I noticed that in the mornings I started singing in the shower again. I was starting to build my life again in a way that was also for me, my enjoyment and wellbeing. No guilt. Life started to flow much better and I felt like I was getting onto my feet again. My daughter was doing well and had a great group of close friends who would stay over sometimes at weekends, and they would start to go out together to friends' parties. I was lucky as there was trust between us and I was able to support her independence in doing the things that she enjoyed. She was enjoying learning to fly, had a part-time job in a café and was well on her way to finding her path. When I think back over that intense period, I realise the important role of enjoyment that carried us through and how grateful I am for friends and family (from afar) who helped us.

There isn't a lot of research about joy, however I found more interesting facts in an article titled 'Joy: a review of literature and suggestions for future directions.' This was written by Johnson (2020), and he quoted the works of many authors in this literature review:

- **Having a disposition for gratitude.** Watkins et al. (2018) gratitude is correlated with increases in the state of joy. The trait of joy correlates with increases in the state of gratitude. They suggest that there may be a virtuous upward spiral in which joy and gratitude mutually reinforce each other.

Meadows (2014) explored the following psychological perspectives of joy:

- **Excited vs Serene Joy.** Excited joy is very intense and involves high energy. Serene joy is quieter and calmer, giving feelings of harmony and unity. Johnson summarises that it is likely that serene joy aims at restoring the body to equilibrium, while excited joy aims at goal pursuit.

❀ **Individuated vs Affiliated Joy**. Individuated joy is experienced as an individual and affiliative joy is joy shared with others. In his study, Meadows found that 70% of the experiences were affiliative and so Johnson surmises that joy is primarily for social bonding.

❀ **Anticipatory vs Consummatory Joy**. Anticipatory joy occurs when the fulfilment of some desire is imminent and consummatory joy occurs when the desire has already been fulfilled.

❀ **Five Dimensions of Joy.**
1. Harmony and Unity. A sense of internal harmony or integration with oneself, and a sense of harmony with the other (including friends, family, nature, etc.).
2. Vitality. Excited joy involves increase in vitality, a sense of energy, potency and aliveness, which activates … Even in serene joy, there is still more vitality than in other emotional states, such as sadness.
3. Transcendence. Consciousness when one senses or has the feeling that he is moving or has moved, soared, or passed beyond ordinary existence. In the midst of a joyful experience, one may feel she has transcended beyond space and/or time, ordinary self-consciousness, the past, or usual personal ego boundaries.
4. Freedom. Joy involves the experience of physical freedom – fluid and free motor behaviours and also freedom of thought.
5. Altered Perception. In experiences of joy, sensory perception may be altered such that individuals experience heightened awareness of colour, depth, touch, etc. In excited joy, colours and sensations seem brighter, sharper, more vivid, and in serene joy, they are perceived as calmer. The perception of time is also altered: in anticipatory joy, the arrival of the thing longed for is felt as imminent; in intense joy, time will 'fly by'; in serene joy, time will seem to pass slowly.

❀ **Joy occurs almost without exception in the immediacy of the present.**
Sometimes it appears that one is in a state of timelessness in which

awareness of ordinary time is suspended, one is not aware of time and feels outside of ordinary time.

Joy vs Ecstasy. Dreyfus et al. (2011) state that ecstasy or bliss wipes you out, joy makes you intensely you. Joy is about your return to fullness.

Johnson (2020) explored the following:

Joy as a Spiritual Fruit. One has a disposition to experience the emotional state of joy (i.e. they have a low threshold to experience it, and they experience joy more frequently across a wider variety of circumstances. They may also experience a subtle and enduring feeling of joy. Additionally, one experiences a deep, spiritual sense of satisfaction, confidence, or gratitude even in the midst of severe persecution, suffering, or sorrow).

Joy and the Imagination. The imagination allows one to take joy in the memory of one who is deceased. In this case the person is made present in the imagination, thereby uniting the individual with their deceased beloved. Similarly, the imagination can also make present a longed-for future situation. In this way, the anticipated joy of the better future turns into present joy, as the better future is inaugurated and made present in the imagination. The future joy turning into present joy creates a motivational state in the individual, in which they receive additional motivation to work to bring that future about.

Joy is the Present Tense. Kierkegaard (1983) believes the whole emphasis should be on the present. And it is the imagination that brings future and past joys into the present.

Joy and the Life Story. McAdams (2001) says joy results from the recognition of one's internal integration, whereby one recognises that one's suffering and sorrow (at the biological and psychological levels, respectively) are consistent with, and vital to, one's life story.

✿   **Literature on Post-Traumatic Growth** by Tedeschi et al. (1998), Nolen-Hoeksema et al. (2002), Updegraff et al. (2000) has revealed that reconstructing a traumatic experience as a situation that was conducive to one's growth, thereby incorporating it into the life story, contributes to an individual's wellbeing and a higher level of functionality (at least in some respects) than before. This raises the question as to whether suffering, as it contributes to post-traumatic growth, may be conducive to experiencing joy more fully.

✿   **Joy and Contagion.** Fowler et al. (2008) believe that happiness spreads up to three degrees of separation, and those who are surrounded by many happy people are more likely to become happy. Johnson surmises that perhaps it is also the case with joy: perhaps the frequency or intensity of joy can spread up to many degrees of separation, and being surrounded by joyful people potentiates joy. Volf (2015) states joy is best experienced in community. Joy seeks company and the company of those who rejoice feeds the joy of each.

In the latter part of Johnson's literature review there is a section headed 'Why research joy?' He states that the answer is very relevant for people who have suffered or suffer with compassion fatigue. He includes Mieder (2009) in an observation of the former president Barack Obama 'repeatedly trumpeted empathy as a quality of character that can change the world' and it was around the time of his presidency that 'empathy' was very much in vogue, and heralded by some as the capacity that had the potential to 'save the world.' Johnson elaborates that affective empathy (the emotional response we have to another's emotional state) has become something of a controversial topic ... Klimecki et al. (2012) describes that affective empathy is subject to compassion fatigue or empathic distress fatigue, whereby aversive emotions experienced in response to another's suffering can be deeply draining and even demotivate an individual from helping the individual in need. By contrast, Johnson states that the existing psychological research discussed in this literature review has shown that joy potentiates action and energises.

Joy provides the motivational resources to act, to intervene, to improve.

That cliché of everything in balance seems poignant here and that joy is an antidote to moving through many difficulties. As Johnson concludes, joy may be the psychological phenomenon that has some of the most potential for bringing about a greater degree of human flourishing and may hold some of the most promise for addressing the challenges of our age. The cultivation of the right kind of joy in the right ways. I believe that this is our must-do task amidst the chaos, fear and worry in the world. I believe it is an antidote.

If joy can help us to flourish, then personally I am all in! Especially when I read that to flourish means to grow luxuriantly – to thrive. Let's face it, joy can be found in the simplest of things and through the imagination! I remember the absolute delight I experienced as a five-year-old opening my gran's silver jewellery box and seeing her beautiful ruby ring. The rubies were the standout amongst her jewellery pieces. I was in awe of their outstanding beauty – there was something luxurious about their colour and depth, even as a five-year-old. It literally made my heart pound, and I can still feel the excitement and joy upon seeing them. When I moved to New Zealand my grandmother gifted me her diamond eternity ring that my grandfather lovingly bought for her. This was a very special symbolic gift, knowing that she was with me forever. Unfortunately, it lost one of its diamonds. When I sold my house, I had a ruby put in its place to further remind me of her. My grandmother was a warm, beautiful nurturing light for me as a young girl – a diamond personified, and I wanted to share her gift with my daughter. I had the ring resized for my finger and had some of the diamonds taken out and made into earrings for my daughter. I felt great joy at sharing my grandmother's diamonds as it was symbolic of sharing my grandmother's light with my daughter.

The Senses

As we know, joy can be found in appreciating the beauty, scent and texture of a rose, the changing landscape of colours in a sunset and hearing the rhythm and lyrical meaning of favourite music pieces. Joy can be found in taking the time to appreciate the simple things through our senses as with tea meditation. The sensory nerves provide us with information about what we are receiving through our eyes, ears, nose, skin, tongue. Tuning in intently to fully see, listen, smell, feel and taste helps us to live more joyfully within our experience of the rose, sunset and music. It is interesting to explore how aware we are of our senses and the ones that we are more tuned in with. When I am trying to move through the jobs on my list, become tired or stressed, my listening or hearing seems to wane. My eyes appear more dominant in terms of what I am the most responsive to. If in a rush, I don't taste my food and don't stop to smell the roses. Appreciating the beauty all around in everyday activities can certainly play a significant role in restoring our energy levels, reducing tension and bringing relaxation.

TASTER ACTIVITIES, TOOLS AND STRATEGIES

1.   **Appreciation (approx. 5 minutes)**
     - From now on each time you write in your journal, note down something or someone that you are grateful for and why.
     - This can be at the start of your journal entry or at the end.

2.   **Connecting your Dots for Joy (approx. 30 minutes)**
     - Look at the framework guide for finding your joy at the beginning of this chapter under the headings of Wellbeing, Belonging, Positive Impact and Fun.
     - Reflect in your journal in terms of where you are at with the above.
     - If there is anything that you want to develop and take forward, transfer it into your Personal Energy Tonic Treasury.

3.   **Johnson's Joy Literature Review (approx. 1 hour)**
     - Reflect on Johnson's literature review covered in this chapter. Is there anything that feels pertinent or that is a standout relevant to you?

- Explore this more in your journal.
- Transfer anything that is resonant, purposeful and meaningful into your Personal Energy Tonic Treasury.

4. **Joy Through the Senses (approx. 30 minutes)**
    - Explore and reflect in your journal about significant times where your senses have brought intense or serene joy, e.g. a scent of an aromatherapy essential oil, the sight of lavender fields, a piece of music.
    - Consider whether your joyful sensory memories have a place in bringing joy now. Can you, or do you want to bring these memories physically into your life again (if you haven't already)?
    - Transfer any of your findings that you may want to take forward in your Personal Energy Tonic Treasury.

5. **Joyful Images Collage (approx. 1 hour)**
    - Go to an op shop and find five magazines that appeal to you.
    - Find a piece of card or paper of a reasonable size.
    - Go through the magazines and cut out images that bring joyful feelings for you.
    - Stick the images on your card/paper.
    - Place your joyful image collage in a place where you will see it.
    - Journal about your experience of this.

6. **Create a Joyful Sanctuary (approx. 1 hour)**
    - Think about items, colours, aromas, photos, images, memories that are meaningful and bring you joy. You may have things tucked away in drawers.
    - Place these items where you can see them, e.g. there may be a beautiful coloured scarf that you love, and you notice that it lifts your spirits. You could hang it on the wall.

7. **Nutrition (approx. 20 minutes)**
   - Consider any new foods to put on the shopping list this week.
   - Take note of any changes you may have made to eating habits, how your energy levels are and what is happening with your fatigue signs.
   - Write any new food items to try in your Personal Energy Tonic Treasury.

8. **Routines and Habits Review (approx. 45 minutes)**
   - Review your diary and energy scores in terms of your new routines, habits and activities – breathing exercises, rest, mealtimes, nutrition, sleep, exercise, playtime, asking for help and enjoyable activities.
   - Make any adjustments necessary in your diary to support your energy levels.

9. **Life Balance Two (approx. 30 minutes)**
   Review the hours that you spend in each of the four areas below.

Weekday

Rest/Sleep	_____	hours
Self-Care	_____	hours
Leisure	_____	hours
Productivity/Work	_____	hours

Weekend Day

Rest/Sleep	_____	hours
Self-Care	_____	hours
Leisure	_____	hours
Productivity/Work	_____	hours

Compare your hours to the first time you did this taster activity in Chapter One. Reflect on your findings in your journal.

10. **The Hand it Over Jar (approx. 30 minutes)**
    - This activity is symbolic of letting go of the things we don't have any control over.
    - Cut strips of paper that you can write on.
    - Find a jar with its lid.
    - On the lid write 'The Hand it Over Jar'.
    - Identify and write your fears and worries about things that you don't have any control over on each strip of paper.
    - As you place the strips in the jar, say out loud, "I hand this .... over to you God or the Universe to take care of ..."
    - Once you have put all the strips in the jar, put the lid back on.

11. **Journalling**
    - Write down any thoughts or feelings about your findings and anything that is happening for you in general.
    - Do you feel that any of the information and tasters will help reduce your fatigue signs?
    - Have you noticed any changes in your fatigue signs, their severity and your energy levels?
    - Can you link any of these changes to adjustments in your routines and activities?

12. **My Personal Energy Tonic Treasury (approx. 20 minutes)**
    In your journal draw your discerning resonant heart as shown below. It may need to take up the full page.
    INNER HEART
    - Write in the inner heart the points that have strongly stood out and resonated in the treasury of information, taster activities/ strategies/ tools that you want to include in your daily life **straight away**.
    - Reflect on whether these things have been helpful towards reducing your fatigue signs and increasing your energy levels.
    - Consult your journal and transfer anything else that is important to you. This may include the adapting or letting go of certain activities

or routines, etc. that you have realised drain you of energy. It could also include ways that you can pace certain activities.

OUTER HEART

- Write in the outer heart the things you have identified that resonate with you and that you would like to change or include in your life **at some point in the future**.

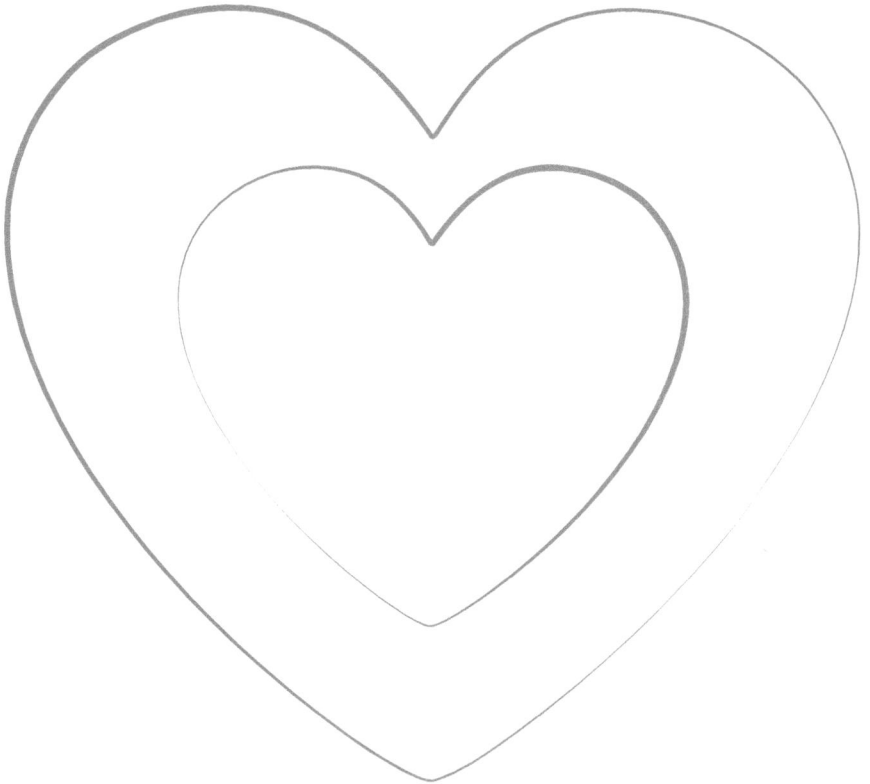

13. Diarise (15 minutes)

- Diarise this chapter's findings from the inner part of your Personal Energy Tonic Treasury.
- You can continue recording your energy scores in your diary so that you can monitor how you are doing.

Congratulations! You have dedicated at least six hours and 45 minutes towards restoring your energy levels through these energy taster activities. This doesn't include your personal journalling time.

References

1. *American Psychological Association*, Definition of 'joy'. Available at: https://dictionary. apa.org/joy (Accessed: September 2024).
2. The Art and Science of Joy, Available at: https://theartandscienceofjoy.com (Accessed: September 2024).
3. Dreyfus, H. and Kelly, S. D. (2011) *All Things Shining: Reading the Western Classics to Find Meaning in a Secular Age.* New York: Free Press.
4. Fowler, J. H. and Christakis, N. A. (2008) *Dynamic spread of happiness in a large social network: Longitudinal analysis over 20 years in the Framingham Heart Study.*
5. Johnson, M.K. (2020) *Joy: a review of the literature and suggestions for future directions.* Department of Philosophy, University of Cambridge, UK P.
6. Kierkegaard, S. (1983) *Fear and Trembling/Repetition* (Hong, H.V. and Hong, E.H. Trans.). Princeton: Princeton University Press.
7. Klimecki, O. and Singer, T. (2012) *Empathic distress fatigue rather than compassion fatigue? Integrating findings from empathy research in psychology and social neuroscience.* In: Oakley, B., Knafo, A.McAdams, D.P. (2001) *The Psychology of Life Stories, Review of General Psychology*, 5, 100–122. Crossref.
8. Meadows, C.M. (2014) *A Psychological Perspective on Joy and Emotional Fulfillment.* New York, NY: Routledge.
9. Mieder, W. (2009) *"Yes, we Can": Barack Obama's Proverbial Rhetoric.* New York: Peter Lang Inc.
10. Nolen-Hoeksema, S. and Davis, C. G. (2002) Positive responses to loss. In: Snyder, C.R. & Lopez, S.J. (eds.), *Handbook of Positive Psychology* (pp. 598–607). New York: Oxford.
11. Tedeschi, R.G., Park, C. L. and Calhoun, L.G. (1998) *Posttraumatic growth: Conceptual issues.* In: R.G.
12. Updegraff, J. A. and Taylor, S. E. (2000) From Vulnerability to Growth: Positive and Negative Effects of Stressful Life Events. In: Harvey, J. & Miller, E. (eds.). *Loss and Trauma: General and Close Relationship Perspectives* (pp. 3–28). Philadelphia: Brunner-Routledge.
13. Volf, M. (2015) The Crown of the Good Life: A Hypothesis. In: Volf, M. & Crisp, J.E. (eds.). *Joy and Human Flourishing: Essays on Theology, Culture, and the Good Life* (pp. 127–135). Minneapolis: Fortress Press. Crossref.

CHAPTER SIX

A Treasury of Sound

Music

Diamond (1980) states that throughout recorded history in all parts of the world, music has been used as therapy. In fact, of all factors that have been investigated, probably none enhances the Life Energy and reduces stress more effectively than music.

The American Heritage Dictionary of the English Language (2024) defines music as:
- The art of arranging sounds in time so as to produce a continuous, unified and evocative composition, as though through melody, harmony, rhythm and timbre.
- Vocal or instrumental sounds possessing a degree of melody, harmony or rhythm.
- A musical composition.

We can use music in a variety of ways to create personal balance and wellbeing. The right genres of music that resonate with us is a kind of nourishment for the soul, physically, emotionally, mentally and spiritually. The word resonance comes up again for the type of music that we may choose for certain situations, feelings, and the type of ambience that we want to create. We can create a peaceful, calm and relaxing sanctuary-like space with our music choices. There could be a soft piece of music that helps with concentration and focus. You may know of music pieces that really help you to let go and unwind in preparation for sleep. There may be pieces where the lyrics really resonate with something that you are going through. These pieces may help you mirror and express your emotions whether it be grief, loss, anger, happiness, joy or excitement. Is there a piece of music that can move us through fear and into courage? There may be pieces of music to energise us. Music is certainly a supportive gift that shouldn't be underestimated in helping to bring us to a state of wholeness and balance.

You may have noticed that the chakra table in Chapter Two has the corresponding musical notes placed beside relevant chakras. Music helps clear what needs to be cleared from our energy field and chakras. Music can also help clear tension out of a room space as well as from us!

In my personal life I can certainly identify with the support that music has afforded me in terms of regulating mood, increasing my energy levels and reducing tension.

Music Creates Ambience and Sets the Mood

In the family household where I grew up with my mum, dad and sister, we had a tradition with Music on Sundays. I mentioned in an earlier chapter that on Sunday evenings we would play the Top 40 charts on the radio. Sunday mornings, however, would also set the tone of an ambient home with the Carpenters, Cliff Richard, Johnny Mathis and the Beatles. Sundays were often a relaxing day for us. Mum would prepare Sunday dinner while the music was playing. It set the scene of enjoying a slower pace and relaxation. When I became an adult with my own family, Sunday morning music also became a tradition.

Music is Energising

As a teenager, music motivated me in the morning, to get me out of bed and have breakfast to be ready for school. Weekday mornings were particularly hard as I didn't enjoy school, and the mornings as a young teenager felt like a lonely time. Dad was usually still in bed as he worked unsociable hours, and Mum was out of the door very early. I started to play my father's upbeat records and Showaddywaddy is what comes to mind. The rhythm and the melody made me feel good when I was feeling reluctant to go to school. I could feel the music opening me up, I could fully feel inside, felt whole, happier and more prepared to go to school. I remember having a buzzy energised feeling, lifted in spirit and like I was firing on all cylinders. It was as though the dislike of school nearly melted away and I was able to face it. The music was literally resonating and clearing the block that I had about school.

My motivation to get to school increased significantly. After discovering that music energised and transformed my mornings, I asked for a Walkman for my birthday. I walked in rhythm with the music to the bus stop and listened to music on the school bus. I was pulsing with energy and my mood and attitude was positive. This vitality started to get me noticed. I realise now that the whole of me could be seen because I was in fact feeling clear and whole. The dance teacher at school selected me to be part of the school annual performances – first performing a dance in a trio, then a duet the following year and then solos in two consecutive years.

Music is an Emotional Support

Music helped me to move through intense anger and rage. This was when I knew my marriage was over. A woman scorned, I reached for the Adele CD. I needed volume and I needed to sing the hell out of her songs from my raging, hurting heart, from the bottom of my lungs and as loud as I could. Letting rip and letting me have it … the anger. Everything out, everything raw, clearing the anger, the rage and making way for the tears. The high-volume part numbing while at the same time allowing the release of raw and real emotion. Adele's lyrics, her singing, with my singing and the volume carried me on a tidal wave. Everything pouring out. All energy centres open, and energy moving out like a tsunami with 'Rolling in the Deep' and 'Set Fire to the Rain'.

I simply did not know what else to do with the floods of emotion in that instance in time. The music supported me, carried me through the torrents, it helped me validate the story and my anger. It brought me to a calmer place. Music also supported me with navigating and functioning through the challenging months to come. It made me realise that I was okay, that I could honour my broken heart, grieve, move through fears, be gentle while building my strength and courage, be functional and know I still had skills and talents, have new meaning in the face of the changes, and start to feel joy. Joy was the important one and music brought it.

The Robbie Williams song 'I love my life' resonated deeply and helped me believe in myself, that I was more than okay and that I had a rightful place in the world, and I could continue to be a great mum to my daughter through this. I read that Robbie Williams wrote the lyrics for his daughter about the ups and downs of life. I guess it spoke to me as the person who was feeling like a child inside as well as it being a great message for my darling daughter.

Thank you for indulging me in reading about my journey with music and how it has supported me. A powerful media! Music is something that can easily be utilised at home, in the car, to bring us a sense of balance and have huge positive ripple effects. It can also be useful if we are worriers and tend to overthink as it acts as a distraction. Using music for wellbeing is a useful self-regulation strategy.

Music Increases Energy and Reduces Tension

The idea of music being a supportive strategy is mirrored by Thayer et al. (1994) at the California State University. They were interested in mood regulation and looked at the effective strategies that people used to make them feel better, increase their energy levels and reduce tension. Exercise was the most successful strategy followed by music as a way of dissipating a bad mood, raising energy and reducing tension.

Below is an energy-tension matrix which can be found on The MEHRIT Centre website. It can help to bring any tension you are holding into your self-awareness as well as energy level ratings when engaged in activities and when resting. You could use this structure using your scale from 1–10 on the vertical energy line (1 at the bottom – low energy end and 10 at the top – high energy end. Have 5 in the middle where the lines cross and fill in the rest of the numbers). Do the same on the horizontal tension line (1 at the far left – low tension end and 10 at the far right – high tension end. Put 5 in the middle and fill in the rest of the numbers on the horizontal line). Mark with a cross as to where you are on these two axes and use this as a feedback and self-regulation tool. Self-regulation after all is a route to calm, relaxation, resilience, energy and wellbeing on all levels.

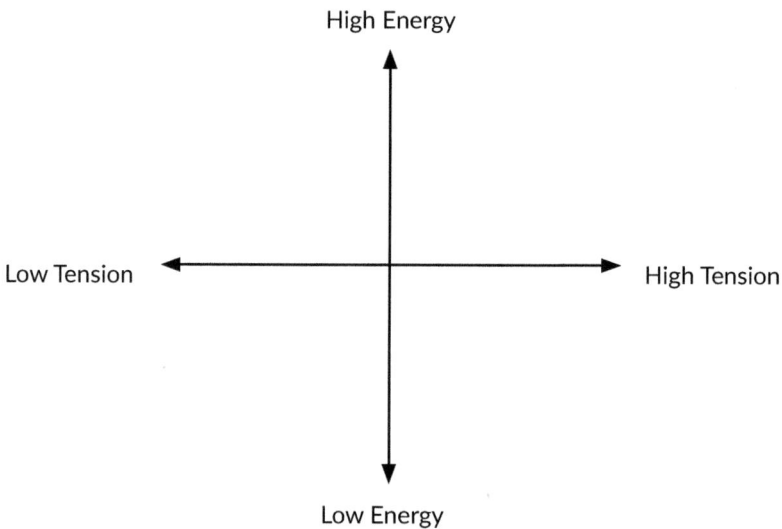

High Energy

Low Tension ←———————→ High Tension

Low Energy

Dr Thayer defined four possible combinations of energy and tension:
- Low energy/low tension: good for sleep and relaxation.
- High energy/high tension: good for physical and mental challenges (sports, getting away from threats, major mental challenges).
- High energy/low tension: alert, yet relaxed state ideal for most daily activities.
- Low energy/high tension: feeling stressed out, irritable, distractible, and lack of energy for doing the tasks at hand.

While this section is written with respect to music and sound, you can probably see that all the subjects contained in previous chapters have been associated with increasing energy levels and reducing tension, i.e. relaxation. Your journey of learning various breathing and relaxation exercises, engaging in enjoyable artistic activities, journalling, clearing space, considering hydration, exercise, nutrition, tea mediations, rest, sleep, play and work have all contributed to looking at preventing fatigue, breaking the cumulative cycle of fatigue and restoring energy levels. You could use the matrix above to get feedback during or after any activity, in different environments and after resting to discern what works for you and what doesn't. Think about how you can adapt an activity, environment, habit, routine, rest period, etc. This tool can be useful now that you are experimenting with and diarising new habits and routines.

Sound

Tomatis (2014) found in his research that high-frequency sounds serve as a vital and necessary stimulant for cortical activity, i.e. the brain needs high frequencies in order to be fully functional. The electrical charge of the brain needs to be regularly replenished. Tomatis contends that the most important function of the ear is to charge the brain through the stimulation of sound. Failure of the ear to provide sufficient recharge to the brain results in fatigue and inefficient mental processes. Ten of our 12 cranial nerves connect to the ear – so the sounds that we hear have a profound effect on our whole system. Dr Tomatis discovered that the ear is intended to hear mainly high-frequency sounds, because most of the sensory cells in the inner ear are accumulated in the high-frequency zone. It is the high-frequency sounds that replenish the brain's energy.

Dr Tomatis describes that unfortunately, most of the sounds that we hear with our mechanised, urbanised lifestyle are low-frequency sounds. Traffic, factories, household appliances, fluorescent lights and even computers put out a low-frequency drone which drains the brain of energy. Notice how different you feel after a day in natural surroundings, hearing only the high-frequency sounds of nature – birdsong, wind and running water. These sounds stimulate the ear in a way that releases latent energy in the brain. The nervous system can then function more efficiently, reducing stress and increasing energy levels.

This is another reason to get out into nature more often as it really can revitalise us, and if we are not able to as regularly as we might want, there are music pieces with nature sounds of babbling brooks, the rolling waves of the sea, the rustling of leaves in the wind and birdsong. More nourishing 'sound food' for thought.

The natural sounds that we ourselves make also affect us, as well as our words. Vowel sounds also relate to each of the chakras. Our heartfelt sound of weeping soothes our soul and cleanses us on all levels. We are releasing our story through the sounds of our tears as we remember and feel. The sound of our laughter also tells a story and moves energy through us. To be with the expression of your emotions through sound is very deeply healing. Releasing through our own sounds heals us physically, mentally, emotionally and is a spiritual balm. Our design is astounding. Consider the simple action of yawning – it allows the movement of air, oxygen/chi to re-energise us, and the 'ah' sound is felt at the heart. Yawn and feel where the sound travels to in your body. Sighing is a sound of release when letting go of a stressful situation and the tension that we have held.

Solfeggio

The Nature Healing Society (2024) describes solfeggio as being the use of sol-fa syllables to note scale tones, that is, solmization. *Merriam-Webster* (2024) defines solmization as the act, practice, or system of using syllables to denote the tones of a musical scale.

Solfeggio is also known as a singing exercise where syllables will be used other than using texts. Every solfeggio tone comprises frequencies that balance our energy anatomy.

Musical Note	Syllables	Solfeggio Frequencies	Corresponding Chakra	
C	do	396 Hz	1st Root	Red
D	re	417 Hz	2nd Sacral	Orange
E	mi	528 Hz	3rd Solar Plexus	Yellow
F	fa	693Hz	4th Heart	Green
G	sol	741Hz	5th Throat	Blue
A	la	852Hz	6th Brow	Indigo
B	ti	Non	7th Crown	Violet

Longdon (2020) in her book *Vibrational Sound Healing* states that interesting studies have pointed towards the calming benefits of tuning music to A at 432 Hz. Longdon describes that this resonance of 432 Hz vibrates with the golden mean phi and unifies the properties of light, time, space, matter, gravity and magnetism with biology, the DNA code and consciousness. That is a very long and powerfully packed sentence. She goes on to say that when our atoms and DNA start to flow in harmony with the spiralling pattern of nature, our sense of connection to nature is magnified.

Apparently, the number 432 is reflected in ratios of the diameter of the sun, the earth and the moon … It is reported that John Lennon's iconic 'Imagine' song was tuned to this frequency. No wonder the combination of the frequency with the lyrical content appears to move people very deeply. This is just my thought upon reflecting. According to the Nature Healing Society, the music we listen to daily is always at 440 Hz in accordance with international tuning standards.

If this topic interests you, it is easy to research the solfeggio frequencies that support us in more detail. Langdon quotes David Hulse (2009), a sound therapy pioneer with over 50 years of experience, who describes in his book *A Fork in the Road* the tones as follows:

396 Hz turns grief into joy, liberating guilt and fear.
417 Hz undoing situations and facilitating change.

528 Hz transformation and miracles, repairing DNA.

639 Hz relationship, connecting with spiritual family.

741 Hz expression and solutions.

852 Hz awakening intuition.

More 'sound food' for thought!

Humming

Graff-Radford (2021) says that humming a favourite tune makes us relax and feel cheerful. She explains that to experience the full benefits of humming, it is suggested you practise a yoga breathing technique called Bhramari. This breathing practice derives its name from the Indian bee, Bhramari. The exhalation in this breathing technique resembles the humming sound of a bee. One of the benefits of this technique is the effect it has on the autonomic nervous system (ANS). When we are tense the sympathetic branch of the ANS activates our body's fight-or-flight response. With this technique the exhalations are longer than the inhalations. This has a calming effect by stimulating part of the ANS called the parasympathetic nervous system. See the bee humming activity at the end of this chapter.

Graff-Radford lists the following possible benefits of humming:

- Reduced levels of stress.
- Lowered blood pressure and heart rate.
- Increased levels of nitric oxide, a molecule that promotes healing and widens blood vessels.
- Improved air flow between the sinuses and the nasal cavity and improvement of the health of your sinuses.

It is fascinating to think that the vibration and reverberation of the sound of our own vocal cords can bring us health and wellbeing! An exciting thought!

The reduction of stress in effect reduces tension held in the body and we enter a more relaxed state and feel more energy.

It is worth looking at the numerous studies showing the benefits of humming and the production of nitric oxide in the body. There is also information that humming supports the detoxification process of the body. It is a big subject, with lots to learn from the simple hum.

Nitric oxide is known to be a bronchial dilator which opens the nasal passages and bronchi in the lungs, improving the uptake of oxygen. It is also a vasodilator, meaning that oxygen can be carried more readily around the body by the blood. This, in turn, makes the mitochondria happy. We know that happy mitochondria means energy production. Nitric oxide is also known to be antiviral, antifungal and antibacterial, all of which support a healthy immune response. Ignarro, Furchgott and Murad (2022) were awarded the Nobel Prize in Medicine for a breakthrough discovery of nitric oxide and how it positively impacts health and longevity.

Singing

Cooper (2020) from The British Academy of Sound Therapy wrote a paper on 'Your Healing Voice – The benefits of singing for health and wellbeing.'

Cooper looked at:
- The scientific mechanisms underlying the relationship between singing and our body chemistry.
- How and why singing can be so beneficial to our overall health and wellbeing.
- The best music to sing along with and how long we need to sing for to feel the benefits.

The Findings:
The full paper can be downloaded from The British Academy of Sound Therapy website, and they summarise the findings as follows:

- Singing alters the hormones and neurotransmitters that boost mood-state and the immune system.
- Adrenalin and cortisol stress hormones respond positively to singing. Adrenalin, the hormone which in excess can cause serious illness, reduces when we sing for pleasure. Cortisol also reduces when we sing; this hormone regulates our metabolism and immune system.
- Dopamine, the happy hormones can release when singing and listening to our favourite tracks, elevating our mood state. They say that every time a song gives you goosebumps or chills, this is a shot of dopamine being released, it's a feel-good neurotransmitter.
- Endorphins are the pain and mood hormones. Singing can release endorphins which can reduce pain and uplift mood. Singing, dancing and drumming all trigger endorphin release whereas just listening to music and low-energy musical activities do not. They recommend that when you sing, get dancing too for a lift.
- Immunoglobulin A (IgA), an immune system booster, supports your immune system by fighting off sickness. Studies have found that singing significantly improves IgA levels.

Benefits of Singing for Mind, Body and Spirit

- As well as the hormonal benefits of singing, the regulation in the breath also helps reduce stress and anxiety. Singing together with others is also beneficial.
- Songs that enhance sustained breathing, tones the lungs and increases heart function by reducing stress and increasing oxygen flow to all parts of the body. There has been research to show certain types of breathing also increases antioxidants.
- Studies show that we are happier when we connect and reach out to others. Singing in groups is a great way to do this. It has to be a no-pressure type of choir or stress hormones will kick in.

In her paper, Cooper states that a study was undertaken by The British Academy of Sound Therapy which explored the use of music as medicine. Over 7500 people took part in the study to find out what kind of music people used to improve their health and wellbeing, how long it took people to feel the effects of the music and what was it about the music that made it so effective. Although this study focused on listening to music rather than singing, it found that more endorphins were released when engaging in music rather than just listening to it. It was found that music with a fast tempo and a driving rhythm and happy or meaningful lyrics are most effective in improving mood-state. It is recommended that you sing for at least five minutes to feel the uplifting benefits of singing. If you are feeling particularly down, then choose a few of your favourite tracks that add up to around 14 minutes to get the maximum sonic vitamin boost!

To determine the therapeutic effects, a questionnaire was used to determine how happy people felt after listening to upbeat music and to which degree the music affected them.

- 32.07% of people felt that they strongly agreed to being happier after listening to the music.
- 64.97% became happier.
- 89.14% agreed to having more energy.
- 64.97% said they laughed a lot more.
- 86.31% agreed to being more satisfied with life.
- 84.67% felt they had a more cheerful effect on others.
- 82.35% agreed that they felt they were able to take anything on.
- 82.4% felt more in control of life.
- 80.06% felt that being happier helped them to make decisions.

Lyrical content with positive or meaningful lyrics are really effective at boosting mood-state. Songs with a driving rhythm are particularly good because they have that irresistible toe-tapping ability! This driving rhythm not only improves mood-state but increases oxygen flow.

In the book *Ikigai: the Japanese Secret to a Long and Happy Life*, the author states that singing in the form of karaoke is a common leisure activity with friends.

Singing and listening to music can be significantly positive in helping prevent and break the cumulative cycle of fatigue, and restore energy flow.

Singing, Sound, Words and Music's Effect on Water

As we know, we are made up of a high percentage of water. The quality of the water in our bodies will impact all the chemical reactions that enable us to create energy. There may be something more to add to this picture as to why singing and listening to music lifts us, energises us and can relax us. It could be the effect that it has on the water inside of us.

While this may seem an 'out there' subject, I want to give mention and space to Masaru Emoto. The businessman, author and pseudoscientist was born in Japan and is a graduate of the Yokohama Municipal University's department of humanities and sciences, with a focus on international relations. In 1992, he received certification from the Open International University as a Doctor of Alternative Medicine.

On his website, Emoto explains that by exposing water to a particular word or piece of music, freezing it, and photographing the ice crystals formed, beautiful words and music create beautiful crystals, and mean-spirited, negative words produce malformed and misshapen crystals. What is the significance? It becomes clear when we remember that the adult human body is approximately 70% water and infant bodies are about 90% water. We can be hurt emotionally and, just like the water can be changed, for the worse physically by negativity. However, we are always closer to beauty when surrounded by positive thoughts, words, intentions and ultimately those vibrations.

You can see how a lot of negative self-talk could negatively affect our waters. I have the image of words being arrows moving into us, through our waters creating wounds.

Dr Emoto believed that words are the vibrations of nature. Therefore, beautiful words create beautiful nature. Ugly words create ugly nature.

https://masaru-emoto.net/en/masaru/

This doesn't mean that if you had a bad day and you are feeling hurt that you bottle up your emotions – writing it out in your journal or talking it through with someone or in fact putting some music on can help. Acknowledging whatever it is, responding to your needs is still important.

If you are interested in reading more about this fascinating subject, I urge you to visit Masaru Emoto's website and see the water crystals in the photograph gallery. He has beautiful crystals categorised into natural water, music, words, photographs and prayer. Masaru also has a beautiful book called *The Hidden Messages in Water* which I highly recommend.

Silence

We have touched on this subject in earlier chapters when talking about complete rest and minimising sensory stimulation, including sound. If we are also able to clear the noise of our own mental chatter, a space is created for another level of quiet and a sense of calm can be experienced. In those moments of quiet with the acceptance that there is nothing to do, nowhere else to be, there is a surrender to just being. Something interesting can occur here in this quiet calm space, as our natural rhythms become apparent. Another layer of sound to the tune of our inner music and rhythm of our heartbeat, breathing along with knowing how our body feels.

Granted it is rare to find silence amongst the busyness in life, within all rhythms there are spaces and pauses. The heartbeat rhythm has its natural pauses between its beats, as does our breathing pattern between the in and out breath, the pauses between the notes of your favourite music or a bird tweeting its song, and the sound of the ebb and flow of the waves. Even the pauses between sobs and laughter, or the kids' shrieks amidst bursts of energy. We can gently listen for the quieter spots amongst the rhythms of life.

TASTER ACTIVITIES, TOOLS AND STRATEGIES

1.   **Steps to Practise Bee Breath (10 minutes)**

Use the energy-tension matrix before and after this taster session and record in your journal.

- Sit comfortably in a quiet place. Take a few slow and deep breaths in through the nose and out through the mouth. As you exhale, feel your body relax.
- Close your eyes or rest your gaze on the floor.
- Keep your facial muscles relaxed, your teeth slightly apart, your lips lightly together and your jaw relaxed.
- Inhale through the nose and then, gently, exhale through the nose, making a low- to medium-pitched humming sound in the throat, throughout the exhalation making a "Hmmmmm..." sound. This should not feel forced.
- Prolong the humming exhalation as long as it's comfortable and you can inhale smoothly with ease.
- Notice the humming vibration on your tongue and the sinus area.
- If you feel agitated, let your breath return to normal.
- Do this practice for about five breaths then return to your normal breathing.
- Take a moment to notice how you are feeling. Notice any changes in your breathing and mood.

https://connect.mayoclinic.org/blog/living-with-mild-cognitive-impairment-mci/newsfeed-post/humming-your-way-to-relaxation/

Write in your journal about your experience and use the energy-tension matrix after the session. If you want to take this taster activity forward, enter it into your Personal Energy Tonic Treasury for this chapter.

2. **Discerning Your Purposeful Music (30 minutes – 1 hour)**

    Music and sound can certainly be a supportive gift physically, emotionally, mentally and spiritually, bringing us to a state of wholeness and balance.

    - Transfer the table below into your journal.
    - Look over the list and choose five desired music effects that stand out the most for you.
    - Identify one or two pieces of music for each of these five music effects that resonate with you.
    - Write the titles of the tracks in the corresponding column. These can either be with lyrics, instrumental, nature sounds or solfeggio frequencies.
    - Plan to use the music tracks this week. At least one piece every day.
    - Journal your experiences and enter any music tracks that were supportive into your Personal Energy Tonic Treasury.

Music Effects	Music Tracks
That creates an ambience of a haven in your home environment	
That energises you	
That makes you feel peaceful and relaxed	
That supports concentration and focus	
That helps you flow with household chores	
That makes everyone in the home feel happier	
That helps you to let go of tension and unwind	

That helps you slow down and wind down in preparation for sleep	
That helps you get out of bed in the morning ... although yes, the kids may be your alarm!	
That resonates with you in sadness	
That resonates with you in anger	
That resonates with you in joy	
That resonates with you in excitement	
That helps you move through fear into courage and strength	
That makes your feet tap and body move	
Others	

3. **Uplifting Daily Sing Song (1 hour)**
    - List seven songs with uplifting lyrics that have a great rhythm, increase your energy levels, reduce your tension, make you feel joyful and get your feet tapping. All of these aspects rolled into a song.
    - Plan to sing one of your listed songs each day, with a goal to have sung them all by day seven. Sing your song for at least five minutes – this might mean you repeat the song to make up the time. You could use YouTube to search the song with its lyrics if you aren't sure of all the words.

- See to what extent you feel energised and the level of tension you are holding after singing your songs. Record in your journal on the energy-tension matrix.
- Do you have favourite songs that increase your energy, reduce tension and make you feel foot-tapping happy?
- Think about activity associations with singing, e.g. doing the dishes, cleaning, laundry and in the shower.
- Transfer any sing-song songs, and any associations you might have with singing during certain activities to your Personal Energy Tonic Treasury.

4. **Energising Hum (40 minutes)**
    - Try humming your favourite tune every day and notice your energy levels, tension and mood.
    - Journal about your experience of humming.
    - Decide if you want to take humming your favourite tunes forward. If you do, place in this chapter's Personal Energy Tonic Treasury.

5. **Nature Sounds (30 minutes)**
    - How will you indulge in listening to nature sounds?
    - In the garden, the park, music nature tracks or another way?
    - Whatever you decide, journal about your experience and use the energy-tension matrix.
    - Write anything that you might want to take forward in your Personal Energy Tonic Treasury.

6. **Nutrition (20 minutes)**
    - Consider any new foods to put on the shopping list this week. Refresh on the information in Chapter Three.
    - Take note of any changes you may have made to eating habits, how your energy levels are and what is happening with your fatigue signs.
    - Write any new food items to try in your Personal Energy Tonic Treasury.

7. **Journalling**
    - Journal any significant experiences this week in terms of what is happening in your life, changes in energy, tension and mood.
    - Transfer anything significant that you might want to take forward to this week's Personal Energy Tonic Treasury.

8. **Routines and Habits Review (45 minutes)**
    - Review your diary and energy scores in terms of your new routines, habits and activities – breathing exercises, rest, mealtimes, nutrition, sleep, exercise, playtime, asking for help and enjoyable activities.
    - Make any adjustments necessary in your diary to support your energy levels, tension and mood.

9. **My Personal Energy Tonic Treasury (20 minutes)**
    In your journal draw your discerning resonant heart as shown below. It may need to take up the full page.
    INNER HEART
    - Write in the inner heart the points that have strongly stood out and resonated in the treasury of information, taster activities/ strategies/ tools that you want to include in your daily life **straight away**.
    - Reflect on whether these things have been helpful towards reducing your fatigue signs and tension and increasing your energy levels and reduce tension.
    - Consult your journal and transfer anything else that is important to you. This may include the adapting or letting go of certain activities or routines, etc. that you have realised drain you of energy. It could also include ways that you can pace certain activities.
    OUTER HEART
    - Write in the outer heart the things you have identified that resonate with you and that you would like to change or include in your life **at some point in the future**.

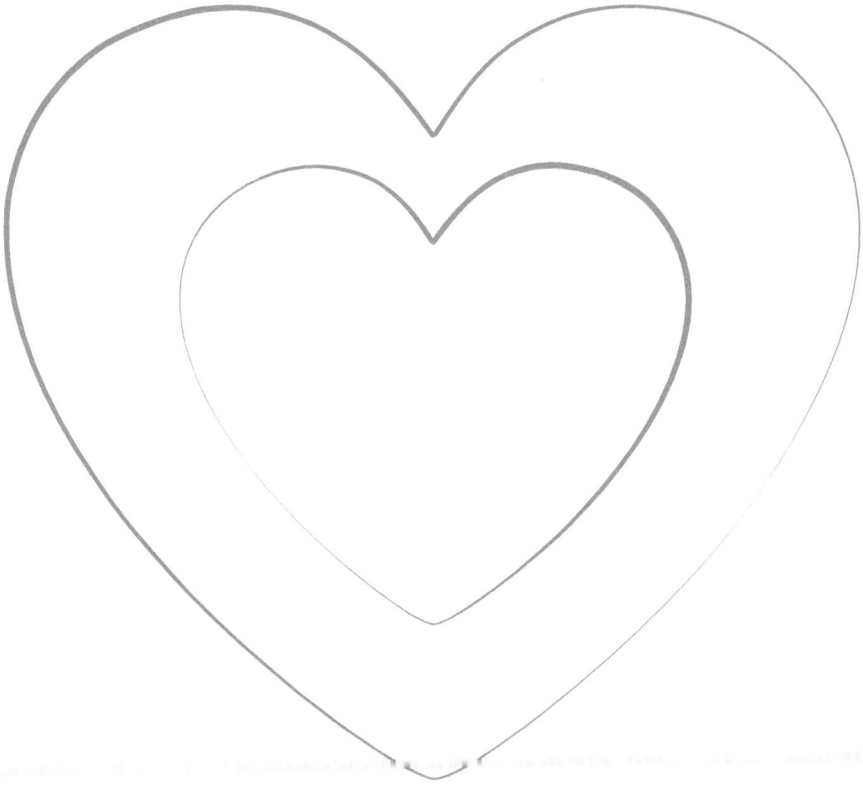

10. **Diarise (15 minutes)**
    - Diarise this chapter's findings from the inner part of your Personal Energy Tonic Treasury.
    - Continue with recording your energy levels to monitor yourself.
    - Decide whether you also want to add in tension scores beside certain activities.

Congratulations! You have dedicated at least four hours and 30 minutes towards restoring your energy levels through these energy taster activities. This doesn't include your personal journalling time.

References

1. *The American Heritage Dictionary of the English Language*, Definition of 'music'. 5th Edition.
2. Cooper, L., MA, MSC. (2020) *Your Healing Voice – The benefits of singing for health and wellbeing.* 30th July 2020, Available at: ICMhttps://britishacademyofsoundthera-py.com/research/singing-for-health/ (Accessed: September 2024).
3. Diamond, J., M.D. (1980) *Your Body Doesn't Lie*, New York: Warner Books, 1980. Available at: https://drjohndiamond.com/ (Accessed September 2024).
4. Emoto, M. (2024) Office Masaru Emoto. Available at: https://masaru-emoto.net/en/masaru/ (Accessed: September 2024).
5. Graff-Radford, M. (2021) HABIT Yoga Instructor *Humming Your Way to Relaxation*, 12th Jan 2021, Available at: https://connect.mayoclinic.org/blog/living-with-mild-cognitive-impairment-mci/newsfeed-post/humming-your-way-to-re-laxation/ pp. 79–80 (Accessed September 2024).
6. Hulse, D. (2009) *A Fork in the Road*. Bloomington, Ind.: Author House.
7. Ignarro, L.J.,(2022) *Nitric oxide is not just blowing in the wind*. Available at: drignarro.com/nitric-oxide-is-not-just-blowing-in-the-wind/ (Accessed: September 2024).
8. Longdon, E. (2020) *Vibrational Sound Healing: Take Your Sonic Vitamins with Tuning Forks, Singing Bowls, Chakra Chants, Angelic Vibrations, and Other Sound Therapies.* Healing Arts Press Pub.
9. The MEHRIT Centre, *Blank Energy/Tension Thayer Matrix*, 8th June, 2023, Self-Reg Tools Series. Available at: https://self-reg.ca/blank-energy-tension-matrix/ (Accessed September 2024).
10. Nature Healing Society. *Solfeggio Frequencies: What are the Solfeggio Frequencies?* Available at: https://www.naturehealingsociety.com/articles/solfeggio/ (Accessed: September 2024).
11. Thayer, R.E., Newman, J.R., McClain, T. M. (1994) Self-Regulation of Mood: Strategies for Changing a Bad Mood, *Journal of Personality and Social Psychology* 1994, Vol. 67, No. 5, 910–925.
12. Tomatis, A. (2014) In: Energy and Sound Therapy – Overcome Fatigue Naturally in Perth, WA. Available at: https://mysoundtherapy.com/au/what-is-sound-therapy/emotional-stress-relief/energy-fatigue/ (Accessed: October 2024).
13. Williams, R. 'I Love My Life', Song Lyrics. Released 20th November 2016.

CHAPTER SEVEN

A Treasury of Meaning and Purpose

I have personally believed since my early twenties that we are all here for a reason, or for many reasons. We all have value and have a special role in contributing to humanity whether it be as a daughter, sister, mother, friend, neighbour, cleaner, musician, support worker, etc. Some of these roles may change and develop through the phases of life. As humans we are all imbued with natural skills, talents, abilities and a passion for something that is embedded within us. We also have core values which we hold dear, upon which we meaningfully build our lives. They help guide us in the decisions that we make.

Core Values

An article titled 'What are Core Values and Why are They Important?' outlines that in the journey of life, we all possess a unique compass, an internal guide that shapes our decisions, defines our character, and ultimately determines our sense of purpose.

At the heart of every individual lies a set of guiding principles that silently dictate the choices we make, the actions we take and the ideals we hold dear. These principles, known as core values, are the bedrock upon which our personalities are built. They are the deeply ingrained beliefs and convictions that shape our identities and define what truly matters to us.

Core values are the fundamental, enduring beliefs that represent what is most important to a person. They transcend cultural, societal and situational influences, serving as a stable anchor in the ever-changing seas of life. They encompass a wide range of ideals, from integrity and honesty to family, adventure and creativity. Core values are not chosen lightly; rather, they are intrinsic to our being and often developed over years of experiences, reflections and personal growth.

Core values can take many forms. For one person, integrity may be paramount, guiding their decisions in both personal and professional life. For another, the value of adventure might lead them to explore the world or take calculated risks in pursuit of their dreams. Family, empathy, resilience, or a commitment to environmental sustainability can all be core values.

Ikigai: Life Purpose / Reason for Being

Many years ago, I came across the concept of ikigai with its corresponding Venn diagram. It inspired me as it resonated and encapsulated something that I innately believed. It also resonated with some of the values and philosophies of occupational therapy which guide practice. Iki = life. Gai = purpose/worth. Everyone's ikigai differs as we have had exposure to different circumstances in life and we have developed in different ways dependent on our values, interests, passions, learnings, skills, talents, leanings and environments.

What it does have in common as stated by Garcia et al. (2017) in *Ikigai: The Japanese Secret to a Long and Happy Life*, is that we are all searching for meaning. They state that when we spend our days feeling connected to what is meaningful to us, we live more fully; when we lose these connections we feel despair. They go on to say that modern life estranges us more and more from our true nature, making it very easy for us to lead lives lacking in meaning. They also emphasise that our intuition and curiosity are very powerful internal compasses to help us connect with our ikigai/life purpose. Follow those things you enjoy … be led by your curiosity and keep busy by doing things that fill you with meaning and happiness. We might find meaning in being good parents or in helping our neighbours.

The Government of Japan website states that ikigai refers to a passion that gives value and joy to life.

Ikigai is said to have evolved from Japanese medicine and the theory that physical wellbeing is influenced by our mental/emotional health and a sense of purpose in life. In an article written by Gaines (2020) titled 'The Philosophy of Ikigai: 3 Examples About Finding Purpose', ikigai is described as being similar to the French term '*raison d'être*' or 'reason for being'. He quotes Japanese psychologist Kumano (2017) as saying that ikigai is a state of wellbeing that arises from devotion to activities one enjoys, which also brings a sense of fulfilment. He also quotes Mogi (2018), saying that ikigai is an ancient and familiar concept for the Japanese, which can be translated simply as 'a reason to get up in the morning' or, more poetically, 'waking up to joy'.

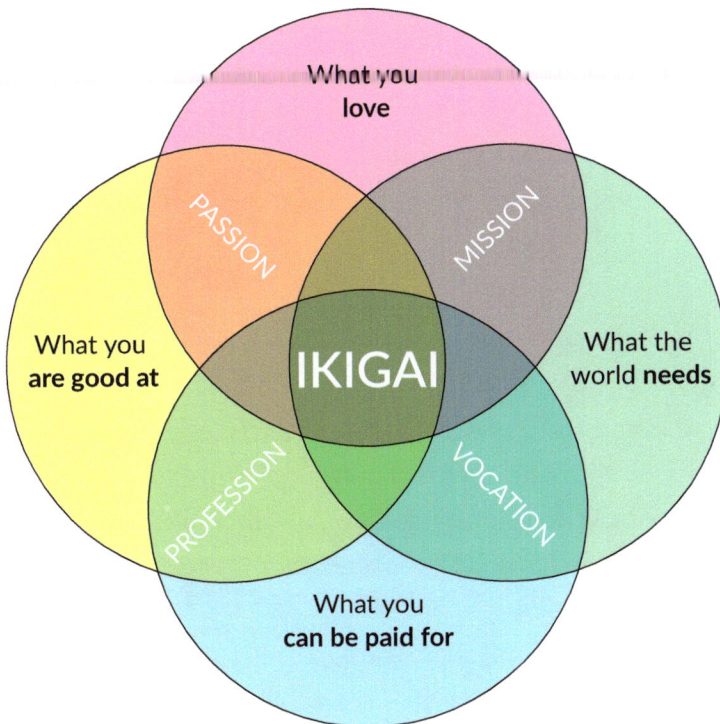

Gaines also states that although it has had some historical shifts in meaning, ikigai has usually been cited as both a personal pursuit and one of benefit to others. Essentially, ikigai brings meaning, purpose and fulfilment to your life, while also contributing to the good of others. He states that everyone has an ikigai – their particular intersection of passion, talent and potential to benefit others. It is only a matter of finding it. The journey to ikigai might require time, deep self-reflection and effort, but it is one we can all make.

Once you discover your ikigai, pursuing it and nurturing it every day will bring meaning to your life. The moment your life has this purpose, you will achieve a happy state of flow in all that you do.

The guidance below is also credited to Gaines and the notes in his article 'The Philosophy of Ikigai: 3 Examples About Finding Purpose'.

You Love It

This sphere includes what we do or experience that brings us the most joy in life and makes us feel most alive and fulfilled. What we love in this sense might be sailing, writing poetry, rock climbing, singing in a rock band, reading historical novels, spending leisure time with friends, etc. What is important is that we allow ourselves to think deeply about what we love, without any concern for whether we are good at it, whether the world needs it, or if we can get paid for doing it.

You Are Great at It

This sphere includes anything you are particularly good at, such as skills you've learned, hobbies you've pursued, talents you've shown since an early age, etc. What you are good at might be, for example, playing the piano, being empathic, public speaking, sports, brain surgery or painting portraits. This sphere encompasses talents or capabilities, whether or not you are passionate about them, whether the world needs them, or if you can get paid for them.

The World Needs It

The 'world' here might be humanity as a whole, a small community you are in touch with, or anything in between. What the world needs might be based on your impressions or needs expressed by others. The world's needs might include skilled nursing, clean water, home heating, election-day volunteers or improved police training. This domain of ikigai connects most explicitly with other people and doing good for them, beyond one's own needs.

You Are Paid for It

This dimension of the diagram also refers to the world or society at large, in that it involves what someone else is willing to pay you for or 'what the market will bear'. You might be passionate about writing poetry or very good at rock climbing, but this does not necessarily mean you can get paid for it. Whether you can get paid for your passions or talents depends on factors such as the state of the economy, whether your passions/talents are in demand, etc.

At the intersection of what you love and what you are good at is your passion.

At the intersection of what you love and what the world needs is your mission.

At the intersection of what the world needs and what you can get paid for is your vocation.

At the intersection of what you are good at and what you can get paid for is your profession.

A 'sweet spot' within this ikigai diagram would therefore involve something you are passionate about, that you are also good at, that the world needs now, and for which someone will pay you. For example, if I am passionate about crisis counselling, am also skilled at it, there is a need for it in my world at the time, and I have several job offers in this field, I might say I've found my ikigai sweet spot.

Gaines states there is a healthy debate about whether the diagram discussed above best represents the traditional Japanese concept of ikigai or a westernised version of it. The Ikigai Tribe (2019) describes ikigai as embracing the joy of little things, being in the here and now, reflecting on past happy memories, and having a frame of mind that one can build a happy and active life.

Whichever the case may be, I feel that it is an interesting exercise to explore. You may of course use it in the way that resonates with you the most. However it is used, I believe that in conjunction with all that has been gained through these chapters, ikigai can further give clarity to our life choices and direction. It gives us meaningful clarity and validation for who we are. Ikigai/ life purpose can help us in planning our short-term and long-term goals.

There is an ikigai exercise at the end of this chapter. Try not to be tempted to do the exercise before you have read the rest of this chapter as the content may be helpful in completing your ikigai.

Resilience

Once we have an idea of our ikigai/life purpose, it encourages us to continue with our passions even when things feel overwhelming. We can choose to focus on what is important and meaningful in our lives, which can prevent us from being carried away with fears and worries.

Garcia et al. comment about resilience and that we all face difficult moments, and the way we do this can make a huge difference to our quality of life. Resilient people know how to stay focused on their objectives, on what matters, without giving in to discouragement. Their flexibility is the source of their strength – they know how to adapt to change and the reversals of fortune. They focus on the things they can control and don't worry about those they can't.

It is worth mentioning here about the Hara energy centre. Hara in Japanese means the centre. I first learnt about developing Hara strength in my Wu Tao training and then as part of Healing Touch training. It is located inside the abdomen just below the belly button. Martial arts training helps to develop Hara, as do breathing exercises and Pilates. When the Hara centre is strong, you can call on physical, mental and emotional strength in challenging situations while remaining calm. We shall explore an exercise to develop Hara strength in a taster activity. The ability to develop Hara strength is a great skill to have as it contributes to our resilience. It is also significant at this point as we have been talking about core values which arise from the core of our being.

Direction and Healing Through Meaning

Ikigai/life purpose could be a valuable guide for finding direction in our lives as women and solo mums. It could be a great route to our health and wellbeing physically, emotionally, mentally and spiritually as it keeps us focused on what's meaningful, purposeful and in line with what we love and enjoy. It gives us some focus for the things in life that we want to set goals for. It also bridges the gap between our self-care and our family life on all levels, which brings immense meaning to our lives.

Shapiro (2006) in her book *Your Body Speaks your Mind* says the original interpretation of the word 'meaning' was to recite, intend or wish. This suggests that without meaning, life is a blank page – there is no story to tell and nothing to recite. But meaning also implies significance and purpose, without which there is no direction and no mission. Meaninglessness can thus cause lethargy, depression, hopelessness and illness. Finding meaning gives direction and motivation, a reason for being that stimulates passion, optimism, strength and wellbeing.

I can relate to Shapiro's theory on many levels. A memory that springs to mind is of my maths lessons at school. Learning how to solve mathematical equations with rules for rules' sake that carried no meaning or purpose, I just couldn't get my head around. I just didn't know what I was trying to work out – and became stuck.

My physics teacher, on the other hand, told the story behind the mathematical equations being worked out. He told the story, explained the process, he drew pictures on the blackboard, and his animated passion for the subject gave meaning and understanding. Interesting that I failed maths but passed physics. The meaning was understood by the verbal and pictorial story which in turn resulted in completing the maths successfully. I needed to connect to the meaning of what I was working out. The equation became meaningful and had context. I had the motivation for learning physics as it held meaning and felt purposeful. Maths, I struggled with – it looked like a sea of numbers that I could not decipher. If I had been assessed I am sure I would have been diagnosed with dyscalculia. Dyslexia with numbers.

This connection with meaning, purpose and direction brings us a natural energy flow which is exactly what we want.

Viktor Frankl's work in logotherapy follows a similar ethos to ikigai. (See the Viktor Frankl Institute of America (VFIA) website.) With a lifetime that spanned most of the 20th century, Viktor Emil Frankl (26th March, 1905 – 2nd September, 1997) was witness to a transformative period in world history. He is most known for being a Holocaust survivor. By the time he entered the concentration camps at 37 years old, he had already spent much of his adult life as a psychiatrist and neurologist, specialising in the treatment of suicidal patients. He had also developed his own psychotherapy school called Logotherapy (Greek for 'healing through meaning'). His lasting contribution has been to the field of psychology, with his recognition of 'meaning' as a central factor in mental health and his advocacy that the psychologist's role was to help their patients find meaning. In the 1930s he worked with teens in Vienna to address the epidemic of teen suicides. Within a year, suicides dropped to zero.

Frankl's experiences in the concentration camps in WWII confirmed his view that it is through a search for meaning and purpose in life that individuals can endure hardship and suffering. He explains that the underlying concept of meaning is the fact that who we are and what we do matters to the world.

'Meaning' often refers to what matters to a person and 'purpose' to one's personal higher calling or a self-driven intent. We do not *push* ourselves towards meaning, but rather we are *pulled* towards it. We do not construct it; it is there, and we intuitively recognise it in a given situation.

On his website, Frankl refers to an example of finding meaning as seeing the shape of a bear hidden in a drawing of a forest with an 'Aha!' experience.

Suddenly understanding something like pieces of a puzzle coming together. When our eyes recognise a meaningful shape in a drawing, it seems to pop out from the background.

The core principles of logotherapy are as follows: Each person is a unique and irreplaceable human being whose existence is characterised by freedom of choice, personal responsibility, and a human spirit.

There are three basic concepts:

- Freedom of Will – We are free to choose how we respond to life and are personally responsible for our choices.
- Will to Meaning – We are motivated to find meaning and when this search is thwarted, we experience existential frustration and feelings of meaninglessness.
- Meaning of Life – We are called moment to moment to answer the demands that life places on us. The focus is not on what we feel we deserve from life, but rather what our responsibility is to give to life. We have the ability and the ultimate necessity to self-transcend in order to improve humanity.

There are vast resources to the human spirit, which is what distinguishes us from other mammals. We are more than just a mind and body; we all have a (non-religious) spiritual or 'noetic' dimension.

The resources available to us include:

- The ability to learn from our mistakes – allowing us to adapt to new circumstances.
- Our sense of humour – putting our failings into perspective.
- Our conscience – giving us the ability to take a stand for things we believe in or against things we think are wrong.
- The ability to love others – helping us move beyond ourselves.
- Our passion for a cause – allowing us the potential to create change in the world.

Meaning can be found through:

- Creations (creating a work or doing a deed) – essentially what we put out into the world.
- Experiences (goodness, truth, beauty, nature, culture, being loved) – essentially what we take from the world.
- Attitudes – essentially how we view the world.

The quest for meaning is the key to mental health and human flourishing. I urge you to have a look at this inspiring website.

TASTER ACTIVITIES, TOOLS AND STRATEGIES

1. **Hara-Building Exercise (20 minutes)**
   - This can be done in a seated or standing position.
   - You can have your eyes open or closed.
   - If standing, have your feet hip-width apart and knees slightly bent with your tailbone tucked under.
   - Place your hands just below your belly button.
   - Follow the pathway of your breath as you breathe.
   - Notice the slight movement of your belly as you breathe.
   - Each time you breathe out, let go of tension and let your belly be soft.
   - As you breathe begin to imagine a golden ball of energy behind your hands in your abdomen.
   - As you breathe in, the ball expands with chi/energy.
   - As you breathe out the ball gets a little bit smaller, letting go of some of the energy, and it starts to feel solid.
   - As you breathe in it expands again.
   - Breathe out and it gets smaller again while shining brightly.
   - Imagine that with each out breath some energy remains in the Hara centre.

- Continue this breathing until you feel a tangible grounded or heavy sensation in your abdomen area and sense of calm.
- Feel your feet on the ground, hear the sounds around you and reorientate to the room.
- Enjoy the feeling of being grounded, energised and calm.
- Journal about your experience and reflect on whether you want to take it forward as a useful practice. If so, transfer into your Personal Energy Tonic Treasury.

2. Core Values (1 hour)

Emily Whitton at the Life Coach Directory UK states that values in life are the things that you think and/or believe are important to you. They are the things that help you guide the way you live and work, can help you determine your priorities, and can even be a benchmark you use to judge if your life is on track and moving towards the way you want things to be. When we are off track, something won't feel right. When we know our values and are living in line with them, we feel on track.

In your journal consider the points below.

- What time in your life have you been the happiest?
- When have you felt fulfilled?
- When have you felt proud?
- What time in your life have you struggled the most?
- With each of your answers, write about what made these times good or tough. Ask who was around you. What were you doing with your days? What values or conflict of values do you think were driving these feelings?
- Next, think of who you admire. These might be people you know personally, family or other role models. Write down what it is you admire about them and consider what values they embody to you.
- From your list of values, create a list of your top five values that you want to focus on.

- From your list of five values, which is the most important and matters the most to you? Ask yourself the same of the remaining four, then the remaining three, then the remaining two.
- Now focus on your top three. Write them on Post-it notes and keep them where you will see them.

Examples of Core Values (this is not an exhaustive list)

Altruism	Empathy	Passion
Appreciation	Equality	Positivity
Attentiveness	Generosity	Pragmatism
Authenticity	Honesty	Reliability
Courage	Humility	Respect
Commitment	Integrity	Self-reliance
Dependability	Kindness	Selflessness
Determination	Loyalty	Spirituality
Efficiency	Optimism	Trustworthiness

Adapted from Emily Whitton's article 'Core Values'

3. **Core Values Vision Board (1 hour)**
    - Go to an op shop and find five magazines that appeal to you.
    - Find a piece of card or paper of a reasonable size.
    - Use crayons or felt tip pens or paints.
    - Go through the magazines and cut out images that resonate with your top three core values.
    - Stick the images on your card/paper.
    - Write or draw anything that comes to mind that reflects your values and how they may translate into your life.
    - You may want to use inspiring quotes about your values.
    - Place your core values vision board where you will see it.
    - Journal about any changes that you may be able to make in line with your values.

- Transfer anything that you may want to take forward to your Personal Energy Tonic Treasury.

4.   **Discerning Your Purposeful Music TWO (30 minutes – 1 hour)**
- Refer to the table in the first Discerning Your Purposeful Music activity in Chapter Six.
- Choose another five desired music effects that stand out the most for you.
- Identify one or two pieces of music for each of these five music effects that resonate with you.
- Write the titles of the tracks in the corresponding column. These can either be with lyrics, instrumental, nature sounds or solfeggio frequencies.
- Plan to use the music tracks this week. At least one piece every day.
- Journal your experiences and enter any music tracks that were supportive into your Personal Energy Tonic Treasury.

5.   **Ikigai (1 hour)**
- Copy the ikigai diagram from this chapter into your journal.
- Reread the guidance notes in turn and reflect on what you love, what you are good at, what the world needs, what you can be paid for.
- Add to the diagram your thoughts based on your self-knowledge, experiences and understanding of the world. It helps you to see where you are in your search for ikigai.
- Journal what your experience has been with this exercise.
- Is there anything that you may want to take forward in the future? Name the things that you might want to take forward.
- Consider if you want to set yourself a goal for the future and any mini goals/activities towards it.
- Transfer anything that you may want to take forward to your Personal Energy Tonics Treasury.

6. **Ikigai Art (1 hour)**
    - When you are happy with your ikigai diagram make it into a piece of art.
    - Transfer your ikigai onto a plain sheet of paper.
    - Use colour, paints, crayons, coloured pencils, etc., whichever form you choose.
    - Place your art where you can see it.

7. **Routines and Habits Review (30 minutes)**
    - Review your diary and energy/tension scores in terms of your new routines, habits and activities – breathing exercises, rest, mealtimes, nutrition, sleep, exercise, playtime, asking for help, enjoyable activities and music/sound.
    - Make any adjustments necessary in your diary to support your energy levels, tension and mood.

8. **Journalling**
    - Write down any thoughts or feelings about your findings and anything that is happening for you in general.
    - Do you feel that any of the information and tasters have helped reduce your fatigue signs, energy and tension levels?
    - Can you link any of these changes to adjustments you have made to your routines and activities?

9. **My Personal Energy Tonic Treasury (20 minutes)**
    In your journal draw your discerning resonant heart as shown below. It may need to take up the full page.
    INNER HEART
    - Write in the inner heart the points that have strongly stood out and resonated in the treasury of information, taster activities/ strategies/ tools that you want to include in your daily life **straight away**.
    - Reflect on whether these things have been helpful towards reducing your fatigue signs, increasing your energy levels and reducing tension

- Consult your journal and transfer anything else that is important to you. This may include the adapting or letting go of certain activities or routines, etc. that you have realised drain you of energy. It could also include ways that you can pace certain activities.

OUTER HEART

- Write in the outer heart the things you have identified that resonate with you and that you would like to change or include in your life **at some point in the future**.

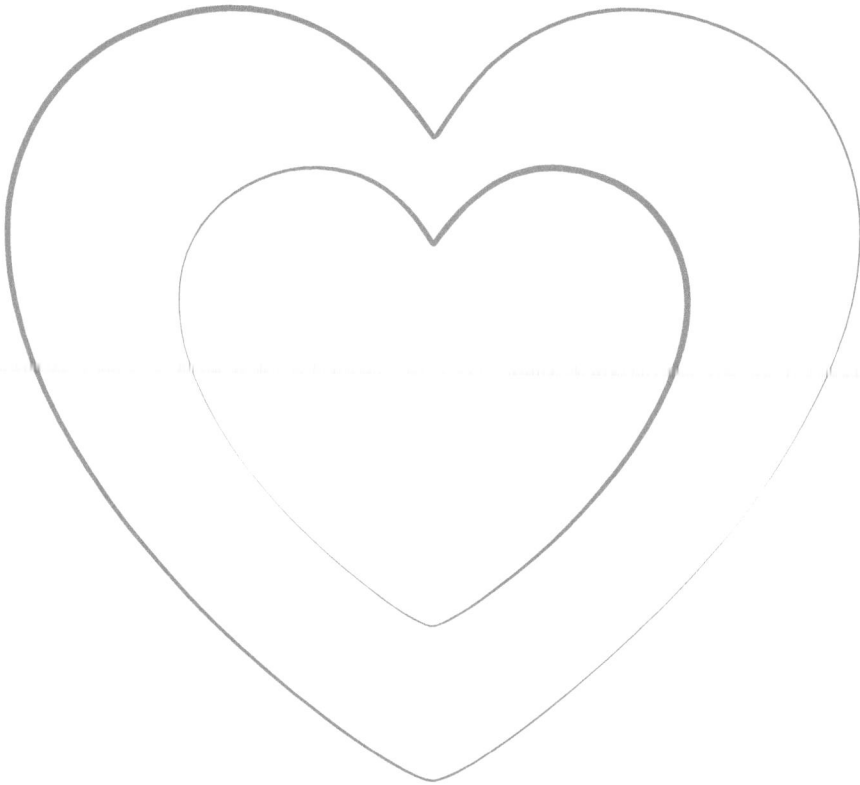

Congratulations! You have dedicated at least five hours and 40 minutes towards restoring your energy levels, ikigai and core values through these energy taster activities. This doesn't include your personal journalling time.

References

1. Gaines, J. (2020) *The Philosophy of Ikigai: 3 Examples About Finding Purpose*, Nov 2020. Available at: https://positivepsychology.com/ikigai/ (Accessed September 2024).
2. Garcia, H., Miralles, F. (2017) *Ikigai: The Japanese Secret to a Long and Happy Life*. Pub 2017 Penguin Random House UK pp. 165–183,
3. Ikigai Tribe (23rd July, 2019). *Ikigai Misunderstood and the Origin of the Ikigai Venn Diagram*. Retrieved 2nd November, 2020, from: https://ikigaitribe.com/ikigai/ikigai-misunderstood/
4. JapanGov, Kizuna Linking Japan and the World. Health and Welfare. *Ikigai: The Japanese Secret to a Joyful Life*, 18th March, 2022. Available at: https://www.japan.go.jp/kizuna/2022/03/ikigai_japanese_secret_to_a_joyful_life.html (Accessed: September 2024).
5. Kumano, M. (2017) On the Concept of Well-Being in Japan: Feeling Shiawase as Hedonic Well-Being and Feeling Ikigai as Eudaimonic Well-Being. *Applied Research in Quality of Life*, 13.
6. Mogi, K. (2018) *Awakening Your Ikigai: How the Japanese Wake up to Joy and Purpose Every Day*. The Experiment.
7. Personal Values. *What are Core Values, and Why are They Important?* Available at: https://personalvalu.es/articles/what-are-core-values-and-why-are-they-important (Accessed: September 2024).
8. Shapiro, D. (2006) *Your Body Speaks Your Mind: Decoding the Emotional, Psychological, and Spiritual Messages That Underlie Illness*. Pap/Com Edition. Sounds True. p. 91–92.
9. VFIA The Life of Viktor E. Frankl, *Meaning from a Logotherapy Perspective: What is Logotherapy?* Available at: https://viktorfranklamerica.com/meaning-from-a-logotherapy-perspective/ (Accessed: August 2024).
10. Whitten, E. *Identifying core values*. Available at: https://www.lifecoach-directory.org.uk/content/identifying-core-values.html#whatarevalues (Accessed: August 2024).

CHAPTER EIGHT

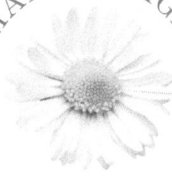

A Treasury of Life Administration

The Treasury and Treasurer of Your Life Admin

The American Heritage Dictionary of the English Language defines a treasury as a place in which treasure is kept. *Merriam-Webster* (2024) defines it as a place in which stores of wealth are kept, and the treasurer as an officer entrusted with the receipt, care, and disbursement of funds. I declare that you are the treasury and the treasurer. You hold and keep the treasure of your energy, who you are, what you enjoy, what matters and is meaningful, and what your purpose is. You decide how you want to store and give your life energy.

Administration is defined by *Merriam-Webster* (2024) as the performance of executive duties. The *Cambridge Dictionary* (2024) defines it as the arrangement and tasks needed to control the operation of a plan or organisation. I would say that life administration is exercising your own authority and will on the choices you want to commit to. These involve your priorities, finding balance in the busyness, putting structure in place with routines, boundaries, self-care, strategies and tools. All these points will be in accordance with what resonates with you personally. You administer your life in the context of what is happening for you, your needs and your roles within your life. Goal setting is also a way of administering your life as you manage it in a meaningful and purposeful way. It is your valuable life as a woman and solo mum.

Commitment and Goal Setting

Merriam-Webster (2024) defines commitment as an agreement or pledge to do something in the future.

Now you know your core values and have an idea of what your ikigai diagram looks like so far, you can choose to set some goals. Your goals will reflect your core values, what is meaningful and purposeful to steer you towards what you want, in realistic bite-size chunks. Having realistic and specific goals can help you to make the commitment without feeling so overwhelmed, at the same time making steady, consistent progress. Goals based on your core values will help with motivation and hopefully be an enlivening experience. Setting your goals as a way of structuring your path with clarity is a great strategy for administering your life.

Reflecting on your ikigai and core values, you can begin to make a list of topics that you would like to set some goals for. You can then review them and put them in priority order considering their value, importance and any sense of urgency. The act of prioritising with regards to your ikigai and values helps to decide which aspects to move forwards with first. This will give focus to goal setting.

BiteSize Learning UK (2024) gives the following guidance for setting SMART goals.

SMART Goals

In the taster activities at the end of the chapter there is structured guidance for setting goals. Have a read here about SMART goals. When you come to setting your goals, be self-compassionate and mindful of your energy levels.

SMART is an acronym for Specific, Measurable, Achievable, Relevant, and Time-bound. The framework is a systematic and simple guide to goal setting that ensures the goals are clear, focused and practical.

Specific

The first step in setting SMART goals is to make sure each goal is specific. A specific goal clearly identifies what is expected, why it is important, who's involved, where it is going to happen, and which resources are involved in its achievement. It answers the 'W' questions: What, Why, Who, Where and Which.

Measurable

Goals should be measurable so there is tangible evidence that you have accomplished the goal. They should answer questions like: How much? How many? How will I *know* when it is accomplished?

Achievable

Goals should be achievable; they should stretch you slightly so you feel challenged, but be defined well enough that you can achieve them. An achievable goal will usually answer the question: How can I accomplish this goal?

Relevant

The fourth criterion for SMART goals is that they are relevant. A relevant goal can answer yes to these questions: Does this seem worthwhile? Is this the right time? Does this match our other efforts and needs? Connecting your goal to a larger 'purpose' makes it more motivating for everybody. Your core values and relating to your ikigai are relevant here too.

Time-bound

Lastly, goals should be time-bound. This means that they have a start and finish date. When you are working on a deadline, your sense of urgency increases, and achievement will come that much quicker.

https://www.bitesizelearning.co.uk/resources/smart-goals-meaning-examples

Examples of SMART Goals: Miles (2023)

SMART goal for writing a book
- ✿ **Specific:** I have an idea for a story, and I want to turn it into a novel.
- ✿ **Measurable:** It should be at least 100,000 words long, and I want to spend at least one hour Monday–Friday working on it.
- ✿ **Attainable:** I am able to dedicate time when the kids are at school for this project. I am an avid reader and writer, so I know what makes a good story and a compelling read.
- ✿ **Relevant:** Reading and writing have always been a passion of mine, which motivates me to become an author myself.
- ✿ **Time-bound:** I'll start writing in the first week of February and finish my first draft by December.

SMART goal example for a side business
- ✿ **Specific:** I will start a side business selling flowers from my garden.
- ✿ **Measurable:** I'll spend at least one hour daily planning and marketing my business.
- ✿ **Attainable:** I used to sell home-grown vegetables, so I already have the equipment, knowledge and reputation to get my business off the ground.
- ✿ **Relevant:** I love growing plants and sharing them with others, plus it would earn me extra money.
- ✿ **Time-bound:** I'll start working on my marketing plans and growing my flowers to be ready for sale by July.

SMART goal for improving emotional regulation
- ✿ **Specific:** I will gain better control over my emotions and feel calmer.
- ✿ **Measurable:** I'll write in my journal each night and rate my mood. Every Friday, I'll review my feelings and thoughts from the week.
- ✿ **Attainable:** Journalling is free, easy, and takes little time. I've been working on mindfulness, so I know I have the awareness to track my emotions.

⚘ **Relevant:** I've started seeing a therapist, and they have encouraged me to set goals related to my wellbeing.

⚘ **Time-bound:** I'm getting my degree and entering the workforce in three months. I want to improve my mood and stress tolerance before then to prepare for my new position.

Here are eight tips for using the SMART goal-setting framework:

1. **Keep it simple:** You may struggle to make large-scale or long-term goals specific enough to fit into this framework. For example, a career change or lifestyle shift may be too nebulous to tackle all at once. If your goals feel too big, break them into more achievable short-term goals to keep you moving forward.

2. **Treat yourself:** Sometimes, you'll need more than just the satisfaction of a job well done. Reward yourself as you reach milestones, giving you something to look forward to.

3. **Goals aren't one-size-fits-all:** The same metrics, time constraints and motivations may not work for every goal you set. Welcome a different approach for work, personal and health goals.

4. **Ask yourself why:** Before you set off on any significant goal, take time to introspect. If your Relevant statement is 'because I want to' or 'because I should', step back and re-evaluate. Determine what you hope to gain, and you'll learn how to better motivate yourself.

5. **Know your limits:** To set attainable goals, make sure they fit your abilities and values. If a task is far outside your range of capabilities, it might be a good idea to set smaller goals along the way.

6. **Write it down:** Ambitions won't become a reality if they stay in your head. Writing out each of the SMART statements reminds you of why you're working so hard. In addition, write out your time frame in a calendar or planner to track progress and minimise procrastination.

7. **Stay flexible:** No plan is perfect. It may become evident that your initial trajectory won't lead to a successful outcome, and staying the

course would only mean wasted effort. Don't be afraid to adjust or reset your action plan if things aren't working out.

8. **Learn from setbacks:** Obstacles provide an opportunity to learn and grow. Take time to evaluate what went wrong so you can become even more effective. But know when to move on. Once you've learned from your struggle, don't continue to dwell on it.

Boundaries and Healthy Relationships

To move forwards with our identified needs, whatever they are, we need to prioritise them as important and literally ring-fence them in our minds and act accordingly. Some of the common causes of fatigue listed in Chapter One are identified as difficulties putting boundaries in place, inability to say no when we need to and want to, struggling to create time and space for needs to be met, overstretching boundaries, and ingrained behaviour patterns such as people-pleasing at the expense of our own needs. We must remember that saying the word 'no' is an act of self-care and self-compassion – being your own best friend. You love and respect yourself for saying 'yes' for what is right for you and saying 'no' for what isn't right for you. Prioritising yourself is important for living your best life. It is also an act of kindling the spirit and saying 'yes' to self-growth. When boundaries are crossed or have been overstretched, we can feel angry with ourselves and others, resentful or even anxious. This indicates a signpost with direction to make our boundaries clear and speak up to support ourselves.

Nash, PhD (2018) is a mental health nurse and lecturer. She states that healthy boundaries are crucial for self-care and positive relationships. In her article 'How to Set Healthy Boundaries and Build Positive Relationships' she offers a guide to setting healthy boundaries. She states that setting healthy boundaries requires self-awareness. We need to be clear about our expectations of ourselves and others, and what we are and are not comfortable with in specific situations. Setting healthy boundaries requires good communication skills that convey assertiveness and clarity.

Assertiveness involves expressing your feelings openly and respectfully. It does not entail making demands, but it requires people to listen to you. Setting healthy boundaries requires you to assert your needs and priorities as a form of self-care. Tawwab, in her book *Setting Boundaries, Find Peace: A guide to reclaiming yourself*, outlines three easy steps to setting healthy boundaries:

Step 1. Be as clear and as straightforward as possible. Do not raise your voice.

Step 2. State your need or request directly in terms of what you'd like, rather than what you don't want or like.

Step 3. Accept any discomfort that arises as a result, whether it's guilt, shame or remorse.

The third step is common for people with poor boundaries, co-dependency issues, or people-pleasers.

Sometimes, adults have been raised by childhood carers who've taught them that expressing their needs is bad and selfish. However, not accepting the discomfort that comes from setting healthy boundaries in adulthood means settling for unhealthy relationships that can cause resentment, manipulation and abuse.

She lists six advantages of healthy boundaries: good mental health, good emotional health, developed autonomy, developed identity, avoidance of burnout and influences others' behaviour.

Examples of Healthy boundaries include:
- Declining anything you don't want to do.
- Expressing your feelings responsibly.
- Talking about your experiences honestly.
- Replying in the moment.
- Addressing problems directly with the person involved, rather than with a third party.
- Making your expectations clear rather than assuming people will figure them out.

Nash says setting healthy boundaries also requires an awareness of different boundaries involved in relationships. Seven types of boundaries are identified:

- Mental boundaries: Freedom to have your own thoughts, values and opinions. "I respect your perspective although I do not agree."
- Emotional boundaries: How emotionally available you are to others. "As much as I want to support you right now, I do not have the emotional capacity."
- Material boundaries: Monetary decisions giving or lending to others. "I already lent you money last week, so not again right now."
- Internal boundaries: Self-regulation, energy expended on self vs others. "I have been social all week. I need the weekend to myself."
- Conversational boundaries: Topics that you do and do not feel comfortable discussing. "I would rather not be a part of this conversation."
- Physical boundaries: Privacy, personal space, your body. "I prefer not to hug people I do not know."
- Time boundaries: How much time you spend with someone or doing something. "I can only stay for 30 minutes."

Asking for help or support in any of these areas can be useful, as goal setting and boundary setting can feel overwhelming if these are new strategies to you. There are also ingrained patterns that we have which can act as a barrier to moving forwards. If this feels like you then coaching or counselling may be helpful. Journalling is also very useful in identifying patterns.

Creativity

Making progress with the above topics creates freedom, space, time and structure in moving towards creating a life that holds much meaning and purpose alongside your values.

In traditional Chinese medicine, the wood element is related to the liver and gall bladder, our ability to grow, express and create. The wood energy is a strong upward and outward movement that allows us to move forwards on our path. It relates to our ability to be responsive to our vision of what we want for ourselves, be able to sense our purpose, plan and set goals towards it. The wood element being associated with the liver is synonymous with the smooth flow of energy. When resting, the blood is stored in the liver and in action the blood is released to deliver energy to the cells. Toxins in our environment, food, drugs and alcohol can create sluggishness and so it is helpful to be mindful of moderating alcohol intake and practising good nutrition.

I include the Chinese medicine information here because it is relevant to how we can become blocked, unblocked and become creatively expressive. When engaged in the creation of this book, for example, I made sure that I took plenty of walk and hydration breaks. It became apparent that my energy flow wanes with sitting for long periods. I begin to hit roadblocks in my creative flow, and clarity and decision making becomes hard. After a walk I can return to my laptop feeling refreshed, energised, and my flow returns.

It is said that the emotion related to the wood element is that of anger. In the western world I don't feel that we are taught how to process and express anger very well. When anger is suppressed, it affects the flow of our energy and forward movement towards our purpose and goals. It needs some form of expression. If we don't express our anger, the energy becomes stagnant or blocked with a sense of an internal pressure cooker simmering away under the surface.

The value of journalling, allowing self-expression, angry tears, talking through with a friend, or a counsellor, painting it out, dancing it out, and any form of physical activity helps the unblocking and expression of anger. You can find your own way of expressing anger that works for you. In doing this, you can decipher the message in your anger and often solutions come to mind. This clears the way for us to be responsive to the message as well as getting back on track with our goals.

I remember a particular situation during my divorce. A great friend held the space while I let off steam about an incredibly unfair situation. I had the mother of all rants; the angry tears and the flow of energy enabled me to ask the questions that I needed answers to. After letting go I felt such a relief from the release. Following the heat of the initial anger, self-compassion and compassion for the situation eased the way forwards. The following morning, I wrote in my journal and was able to compose an email that was honest and firm, asking relevant questions regarding the situation. Within a few minutes of the email being sent, I had a positive reply. The problems were resolved quickly with clarity about an effective solution and way forwards. I found the process nothing short of miraculous. If I had suppressed the emotion, I couldn't gain clarity, which would result in no flowing energy. Expression and freeing the energy equals clarity and creating a way forwards.

As I mentioned earlier, the wood element is associated with the liver and the gall bladder – they work as a supporting mechanism with each other. It is said that the energy of the gall bladder helps us with clarity of direction, decision making and flexibility of thinking when reasoning about how we want to move forwards.

You can now pave your way to creating your ikigai at your own pace, in your way. The important thing is to enjoy the journey. Through gentleness with yourself/self-compassion you will gain strength. Goals can always be adapted if needed. Goals are flexible. The world needs people who can connect with their joy, their passion, natural skills and abilities towards a purpose. We need it individually for wellbeing, our families need it, and society needs it. A win, win, win!

TASTER ACTIVITIES, TOOLS AND STRATEGIES

1. **Priorities (45 minutes)**
    - Reflect on your ikigai and core values then make a list of topics you would like to set some goals for.
    - Put your topics list for your goals in priority order, considering their value, how important and meaningful they are, and any sense of urgency.
    - Choose your top priority topic.

2. **SMART Goal Setting (1hour)**
   - Have a play with setting goals in your journal for your priority topic that you selected.
   - When setting your goals be self-compassionate and mindful of your energy levels.
   - You can use the template below to guide you.
   - Use the examples in the chapter for a reference point.
   - You might even change your priority topic, having gone through the process.

SMART GOALS

SPECIFIC

A specific goal clearly identifies what is expected, why it is important, who's involved, where it is going to happen, and which resources are involved in its achievement. It answers the 'W' questions: What, Why, Who, Where and Which.

_____

_____

_____

_____

_____

_____

MEASURABLE

Goals should be measurable so there is tangible evidence that you have accomplished the goal. They should answer questions like: How much? How many? How will I know when it is accomplished?

_____

_____

_____

_____

_____

_____

_____

ACHIEVABLE

Goals should be achievable; they should stretch you slightly so you feel challenged, but defined well enough that you can achieve them. An achievable goal will usually answer the question: How can I accomplish this goal?

_____

_____

_____

_____

_____

_____

RELEVANT

A relevant goal can answer yes to these questions: Does this seem worthwhile? Is this the right time? Connecting your goal to a larger 'purpose', your core values and ikigai.

_____

_____

_____

_____

_____

_____

TIME- BOUND

This means your goals have a start and finish date. When you are working on a deadline, your sense of urgency increases, and achievement will come that much quicker.

_____

_____

_____

_____

_____

_____

_____

3.   **Smart Statement and Commitment Statement (30 minutes)**

- Once you have crafted your SMART statement, write it on a piece of paper and place it where you can see it.
- Write out your time frame in a calendar or planner along with the tasks to track progress and minimise procrastination.
- This process can be repeated with your next priority topic when the time is right for you in the future.

SMART STATEMENT/GOAL

Review your answers and bring them together to make a goal statement.

_____

_____

_____

_____

_____

_____

_____

_____

COMMITMENT STATEMENT

Agreement and pledge to yourself.

I .... *Your Name* .... agree to pledge my commitment to this goal. I have faith that I can make progress towards it. If circumstances change, I will adapt the goal so that it is still achievable. I will continue to self-care for my energy levels while moving forwards with this goal. I know that I matter, and this goal is important to me. I move forwards with my goal in a self-compassionate and gentle way.

.... *Your Signature* ....

---

4.   **Task List for SMART goals (15 minutes)**
   - List all the tasks in your journal that are related to your goals.
   - Start putting them in your diary, e.g. any research you need to do or telephone calls, etc.

5.   **Boundary Setting (30 minutes)**
   - Reflect on the section about boundaries and relationships in your journal.
   - Ask yourself whether you will need to put any boundaries in place for your goals and self-care needs to be met.
   - If you attend to putting boundaries in place, journal about how that went, how you felt and if you were heard.

6.   **Vision Board (45 minutes)**
   - Find a piece of card or paper of a reasonable size.
   - Use crayons or felt tip pens or paints and pictures from magazines.
   - Create a collage that reflects your SMART goal statement and how it will positively impact your life and others.
   - You may want to use inspiring quotes.

- Place your vision board in a place where you will see it.

7. **Creativity Reflection (30 minutes)**
    - Reflect on the creativity section and whether there is anything that resonates there or any standout points.
    - Consider whether there is anything that you may want to take forward. If so, transfer it to your Personal Energy Tonic Treasury.

8. **Journalling**
    - Write down any thoughts or feelings about your findings and anything that is happening for you in general.
    - Do you feel that any of the information and tasters have helped reduce your fatigue signs, energy and tension levels?
    - Can you link any of these changes to adjustments you have made to your routines and activities?

9. **My Personal Energy Tonic Treasury (20 minutes)**
    In your journal draw your discerning resonant heart as shown below. It may need to take up the full page.
    INNER HEART
    - Write in the inner heart the points that have strongly stood out and resonated in the treasury of information, taster activities/ strategies/ tools that you want to include in your daily life **straight away**.
    - Reflect on whether these things have been helpful towards reducing your fatigue signs, increasing your energy levels and reduce tension.
    - Consult your journal and transfer anything else that is important to you. This may include the adapting or letting go of certain activities or routines, etc. that you have realised drain you of energy. It could also include ways that you can pace certain activities.
    OUTER HEART
    - Write in the outer heart the things you have identified that resonate with you and that you would like to change or include in your life **at some point in the future**.

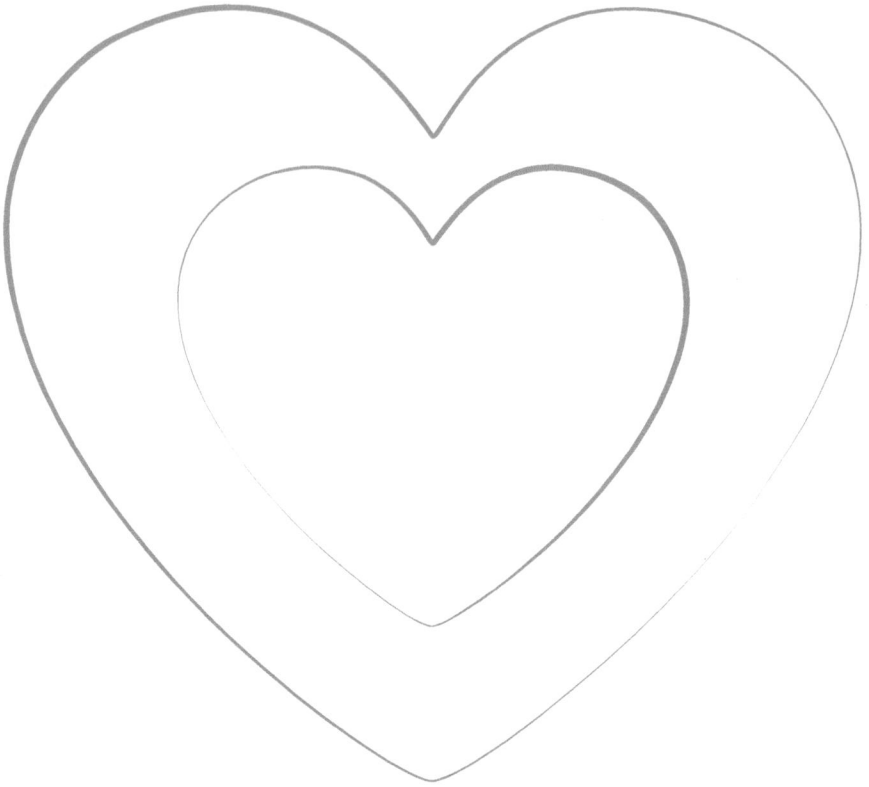

10. Diarise (15 minutes)

Diarise anything from this week's findings from the inner part of your Personal Energy Tonic Treasury.

Congratulations! You have dedicated at least four hours and 50 minutes towards restoring your energy levels and creating your future through these energy taster activities. This doesn't include your personal journalling time.

References

1. *The American Heritage Dictionary of the English Language*, Definition of 'treasury'. 5th Edition.
2. BiteSize Learning UK. *SMART goals: a guide to setting goals that matter*. Available at:

https://www.bitesizelearning.co.uk/resources/smart-goals-meaning-examples (Accessed: September 2024).

3. Miles, M. (2023) *10 SMART goal examples for your whole life.* Available at: https://www.betterup.com/blog/smart-goals-examples 27th July 2023 (Accessed September 2024).

4. Nash, J., PhD. (2018) *How to Set Healthy Boundaries & Build Positive Relationships* 5th Jan 2018. Available at: https://positivepsychology.com/great-self-care-setting-healthy-boundaries/ (Accessed: September 2024).

5. Tawwab, N. G. (2021). Set boundaries, find peace: A guide to reclaiming yourself. Little, Brown Book Group.

CHAPTER NINE

A Treasury of Support

This chapter holds a resource of contacts as a support network for you. This book was born in New Zealand and therefore the support contact networks listed are NZ based. You can use this list as a subject template to research supportive contacts in your country of residence.

Sometimes we need a bit of extra support at difficult times due to all kinds of reasons. Support is to keep us from weakening or failing; give confidence or comfort to, according to *The American Heritage Dictionary of the English Language.*

As we know, as human beings we have physical, emotional, mental and spiritual aspects of ourselves that show up as needs. These are our signposts. When self-aware, we are able to recognise a need that is difficult to manage and fulfil. We are self-compassionate in accepting that support is needed, and when we ask, we are likely to receive help from others. We can do our best and take responsibility for fulfilling our needs, as well as recognising when we need to ask for support.

We mustn't forget that our wellbeing also requires a sense of belonging through social connectivity. While this subject has been mentioned when discussing topics such as play, work and enjoyment, it is worth mentioning again. Looking at the meaning of social connectedness and belonging can help us to see if we have needs in these areas that can be sought to be fulfilled

Social Connectedness: The opposite of loneliness, a subjective evaluation of the extent to which one has meaningful, close, and constructive relationships with others (i.e., individuals, groups, and society). *O'Rourke*

Belonging: A feeling of being happy or comfortable as part of a particular group and having a good relationship with the other members of the group because they welcome you and accept you. *Cambridge Dictionary*

Garcia and Miralles state in the *Ikigai* book that part of the lifestyle of the people in Ogimi, Japan is that they all belong to a neighbourhood association, where they feel cared for like a family member. This is part of their secret to wellness. We can research what clubs or organisations are out there that are in line with our interests, and what we value and enjoy.

6 Types of Support

Emotional Support

Emotional support is about demonstrating empathy and understanding, and offering reassurance and encouragement, especially during difficult times. It involves being an empathetic listener, validating others' feelings, and providing a comforting presence, which are crucial in nurturing mental and emotional wellbeing.

Financial Support

This type of support refers to providing monetary assistance to alleviate financial burdens. It can come directly through financial aid or indirectly via advice and guidance on budgeting and financial planning. Financial support helps relieve stress associated with financial insecurities, contributing to a more stable environment for individuals to thrive in.

Physical Support

Physical support includes hands-on assistance with activities of daily living, mobility, and other physical needs. This kind of support is vital for individuals with physical limitations or those recovering from illness, helping them maintain independence and quality of life.

Social Support

Facilitating a sense of belonging and companionship, social support involves spending quality time together, engaging in social activities, or being a reliable friend or family member. Strong social networks are foundational to mental health, providing individuals with a sense of community and connection.

Practical Support

Practical support consists of offering tangible assistance with day-to-day tasks and challenges. This can range from helping with paperwork and offering transportation to assisting in home repairs or organisation, easing the daily burdens on individuals and helping them focus on their wellbeing.

Informational Support

Providing advice, sharing knowledge, or offering resources to help individuals make informed decisions is key to informational support. This encompasses educating others, mentoring or guiding them through complex processes or decisions, and empowering individuals with the information they need to navigate life's challenges effectively.

Human Integrated Performance

Support Network Task

- Consider whether you have any gaps in the above types of support and make a list accordingly.
- Remember to be self-compassionate.
- If you have some gaps in support, remember that almost everyone needs support at some time in their lives. Be gentle.

☆ Scan the Supportive Contact list below and see if any fit what you need.

☆ Search the internet for any other groups or organisations that may be of benefit.

☆ Write down exactly what you need help with.

☆ Take a deep breath and pick up the phone and ask for a chat or an appointment.

Below I have compiled a list of supportive contacts who may be able to help with practical and professional support if needed.

Supportive Contacts:

Healing Touch New Zealand

Healing Touch was developed by a nurse in Colorado (Janet Mentgen). It has comprehensive and rigorous training, a foundation of core values, formal documentation requirements and a code of ethics/standards of practice that guide the energetic and holistic practice of healing touch.

☆ Healing Touch is a relaxing, nurturing energy therapy that uses light, gentle touch to clear, balance and restore flow to the human energy system assisting with physical, mental, emotional and spiritual wellbeing.

☆ A compassionate approach, listening from the heart and prioritising needs together.

☆ Specific techniques are used to promote balance to the energy anatomy, restoring energy flow.

☆ Useful techniques can be used to promote deep relaxation, reduce anxiety, tension, stress and fatigue, help with depression, increase energy and promote sleep.

☆ Techniques can be used to reduce pain, headaches, migraines, provide support in major life transitions and challenges, support post trauma, deal with unresolved emotions, support decision making and forgiveness.

✿ Strengthens the immune system, helps to release emotional/spiritual pain/grief, as well as promoting clarity, calmness, and quiet of the mind.

✿ An ideal support for solo mums. It is also ideal for a mum if she has endured violence as techniques can be implemented as mostly hands off (minimal physical contact) if required.

www.healingtouchnz.com to find a practitioner in your area.

Birthright.org.nz

The home page of the website states that they offer a range of social services for the children and parents of families led by one person. Their goal is nurtured, resilient and inspired children and families. The support they provide is confidential, non-judgemental, friendly and in most cases free of charge.

✿ Social work support and counselling for children, families and whānau.

✿ Parent education programmes.

✿ Budgeting advice.

✿ Referrals to recognised agencies for specialist services.

✿ Parent networking opportunities.

✿ Self-esteem programmes for children.

✿ Some financial assistance with school requirements and holiday camps.

✿ Practical assistance with clothing supplies and household items.

✿ Access to resources and information.

✿ Advocacy Support.

✿ Help you connect with your community.

Tel: 0800 457 146. https://birthright.org.nz/our-services

Lifeline (Presbyterian Support Northern)

Lifeline works in partnership with Parent Help for parent and family support.

0800 543 354 or text 'Help' to 4357. Free service, available 24 hours a day, 365 days a year. https://www.lifeline.org.nz/

TAUTOKO Suicide Crisis Helpline 24 hours a day, seven days a week. 0508 828 865 https://www.lifeline.org.nz/services/suicide-crisis-helpline

Parent Helpline

Parent Helpline offers compassionate, friendly, non-judgemental support and advice on all parenting issues – no issue is too big or too small.

Some of the issues they can help with include:

- Disrespectful and out-of-control behaviour
- Sibling rivalry
- Solo parenting
- Refusing to go to school
- Blended families
- Posting on social media
- Boundaries
- Aggression and anger issues
- Sexting
- Technology and device use
- Abuse
- Anxiety and depression
- Bullying
- Tantrums
- Self-harming

Lifeline works in partnership with Parent Help for parent and family support.

0800 568 856 https://www.parenthelp.org.nz/

PlunketLine

A free parent helpline and advice service available to all families, whānau and caregivers 24 hours a day, seven days a week.

- ✿ You don't need to be a Plunket client to use PlunketLine.
- ✿ When you call PlunketLine your call will be answered by a Plunket nurse, who can give you advice and information on parenting issues and your child's health and wellbeing.
- ✿ You can also access free online specialist support with breastfeeding and sleep through PlunketLine.

0800 933 922 Calls are free including from cell phones

https://www.plunket.org.nz

Work and Income

0800 559 009 Mon – Fri, 7 am to 6 pm. Sat, 8 am to 1 pm.

https://www.workandincome.govt.nz

Samaritans Aotearoa New Zealand

- ✿ Confidential, non-judgemental and non-religious support.
- ✿ If you are experiencing loneliness, depression, despair, distress or suicidal feelings, call 0800 72 66 66 now.
- ✿ Samaritans operates a 24/7 crisis helpline. Our phones are operated by volunteers from the community for the community. We receive no direct government funding.
- ✿ "There is no greater agony than bearing an untold story inside you." Maya Angelou.

0800 72 66 66 Free lhttps://www.samaritans.org.nz

Youthline

- Free, confidential and non-judgemental telephone counselling service, available 24/7, 365 days a year for all young people.
- Youthline is a 'with youth, for youth' organisation that supports young people throughout Aotearoa New Zealand. They have been providing support to Kiwis aged between 12–24 years for more than 50 years.
- Youthline is here to support all young people – this includes young people who are struggling (with their mental health or other issues), as well as young people who want to learn, grow and give back to their community.
- Youthline offers a free helpline service (text, phone, webchat and email), free face-to-face counselling services, youth mentoring, programmes in schools and communities to help people grow and develop.

0800 376 633 or text 234. https://youthline.co.nz/about-us/

Parenting Place

- 30 years of supporting parents in Aotearoa.
- Parenting courses, one-on-one parent coaching, parenting talks, media interviews, articles and online resources to inspire, equip and support thriving and connected whānau throughout Aotearoa.
- They believe that every family can benefit from good parenting information, encouragement and nurturing. And that healthy, loving families can transform communities.
- They support anyone raising a child, including parents, caregivers, grandparents, aunties, uncles, guardians and foster carers.

0800 535 659 or 09 524 0025 https://parentingplace.nz

KIWI Families

- A website with free tips, tools and advice from some of the best New Zealand parenting experts.
- Advice and wellbeing
- Pregnancy and birth
- Topics by age
- Lifestyle

https://www.kiwifamilies.co.nz

Loneliness NZ

- Providing comprehensive information and support on conquering loneliness.
- Self-Help Resources: Providing resources for those experiencing loneliness.
- Counselling and Coaching: Providing interventions for those experiencing prolonged or chronic loneliness.
- Preventative Skills Training: Up-skilling individuals in the prevention of loneliness through group coaching sessions.
- Collaborative Efforts: Working with researchers, other organisations, government and media to address loneliness.

https://loneliness.org.nz

References

1. *The American Heritage Dictionary of the English Language*, Definition of 'support'. 5th Edition.
2. Garcia, H., Miralles, F. (2017) *Ikigai: The Japanese Secret to a Long and Happy Life.* Pub Penguin Random House 2017.

3.   Human Integrated Performance. *What are the 7 types of support?* Available at: https:// yeghip.com/faq/what-are-the-7-types-of-support/ (Accessed: September 2024).

4.   O'Rourke, H. M. and Sidani, S. (2017) Definition, determinants, and outcomes of social connectedness for older adults: A scoping review. *Journal of Gerontological Nursing*, 43(7), 43–52.

CHAPTER TEN

A Treasury of Celebration and Flourishing

The Collins English Dictionary (2024) defines celebration as a special enjoyable event that people organise because something pleasant has happened or because it is someone's birthday or anniversary. The celebration of something is praise and appreciation which is given to it.

This final chapter is a celebration of what you have achieved so far in completing the previous chapters.

You have explored nine treasuries:
- A Treasury of Fatigue Awareness and Self-Compassion
- A Treasury of Life Energy
- A Treasury of Energy Tonics
- A Treasury of the Big Four
- A Treasury of Joy
- A Treasury of Sound
- A Treasury of Meaning and Purpose
- A Treasury of Life Administration
- A Treasury of Support

Through completing these chapters, you will have:
- Discerned your personal treasury of energy tonics.

- Hopefully moved through fatigue (reduced the severity of your symptoms) to improved energy levels and restoration with self-compassion.
- More enjoyment in your life.
- Found your core values that can guide decisions in your life.
- Started finding your ikigai that brings meaning and purpose to yourself and the world.
- Put structure in place to guide you with meaningful and purposeful goals.
- Realised any support that you may need and asked for help.
- Experienced a natural positive ripple effect through to your family life.

To flourish is to find fulfilment in our lives, says Seligman (2011), accomplishing meaningful and worthwhile tasks, and connecting with others at a deeper level – in essence, living the 'good life'.

Seligman explains there are five factors that contribute to flourishing. These are positive emotions, engagement, relationships, meaning and accomplishments.

Positive psychologist Professor Soots (2015) describes flourishing as the product of the pursuit and engagement of an authentic life that brings inner joy and happiness through meeting goals, being connected with life passions, and relishing in accomplishments through the peaks and valleys of life.

Moving through your process in the treasuries has led you to this point. A cause for celebration in your achievement, moving through the gateway to flourishing. With the embracing of self-compassion, it is hoped that you have enjoyed celebrations small and large through your achievements.

Flourishing requires ongoing nurturing. The nurturing of continued self-compassion and attending needs, restoration, enjoyment, living by core values, living meaningfully and purposefully (ikigai), setting goals and growing ourselves and our relationships.

My wish is for you to flourish as a wonderful woman, daughter, mum, homemaker, friend, neighbour, community member, colleague, artist, gardener and anything that you do. My hope is that there has been a shift from low energy to restoration, high energy and flourishing. You are important, you are worth it. It's your birthright to flourish. Solo Mums Matter. Forget You Not.

So, I warmly sign off with some celebratory activities for thought and three ongoing tasks for flourishing!

Celebratory Activities:

1. **Your Personal Energy Tonic Treasury: A Piece of Art**
   - Look back at each of your Personal Energy Tonic Treasuries.
   - Make a piece of art.
   - On a large sheet of paper draw yourself one large heart.
   - Put all the items that you have placed in your Personal Energy Tonic Hearts inside this heart.
   - Place your core values in your heart.
   - Place your ikigai in your heart.
   - Place your SMART Goal statement in your heart.
   - Place your supports in your heart.

2. **Compassionate Reflections**
   - As you look at your piece of art, take some time to reflect on what you have achieved.
   - Feel compassion for yourself and thank yourself for moving through this adventure.
   - What have been the most important changes you have made?
   - What barriers have you moved through?
   - How did you move through the barriers?
   - Feel a sense of thankfulness for allowing yourself to move forwards, even when there have been uncomfortable feelings.
   - What strengths did you use?
   - Who has helped you along the way?
   - What did you enjoy the most?

3. **Plan a Celebration**
    - Plan a fun celebration either with others, family or yourself.
    - Celebrate in a way that nourishes you physically, emotionally, mentally, and lifts your spirits.
    - Be sure to make a statement honouring that this is a special celebration of...............
    - Enjoy your special celebration.
    - Take photos to remember the occasion.
    - Place the photo where you will see it regularly.
    - Journal your experience.

Administer Your Life from Your Treasury

- Be self-compassionate.
- Be aware of your fatigue signs and triggers.
- Be aware of your energy and tension levels.
- Respect the big four – sleep, rest, play, work.
- Be responsive with your energy tonics.
- Find joy.
- Schedule enjoyable activities.
- Resonate with sound.
- Live according to your values.
- Find meaning and purpose – ikigai.
- Set your goals and boundaries.
- Ask for support when needed.
- Celebrate achievements big and small.

Flourishing Energy Tonic Treasury

- Look back over your Personal Energy Tonic Treasury Hearts.
- Focus on the items that you placed in the outer edge of your heart for change or inclusion in your life for the future.

❀ List them all on a sheet of paper.

❀ Place them in priority order in terms of whether they are in line with your values and ikigai, will increase your energy levels, reduce tension, and bring enjoyment. You may decide to let some of the items go.

❀ On a sheet of paper draw a large discerning resonant heart as shown below. It may need to take up the full page.

❀ Put the item that is your number one priority in the centre heart.

❀ Put the remaining items in the outer heart with their number priority next to each.

❀ As you attend the priority in the centre, put a tick next to it and add the number two priority in the centre, and so on.

❀ Pace yourself as you move through the priorities.

❀ Add anything new and significant either into the centre for integration now or on the outer edge for later.

❀ Keep flowing with this process for keeping track and for your flourishing.

SMART Goal for Flourishing

Continue to pace the setting of your goals in line with your core values and ikigai.

References

1. Seligman, M. E. P. (2011) *Flourish: A Visionary New Understanding of Happiness and Well-being.* New York City, NY: Atria Books.
2. Soots, L. (2015) (n.d.) *Flourishing.* March 2015 The Positive Psychology People. Available at: http://www.thepositivepsychologypeople.com/flourishing (Accessed: September 2024).

SOLO MUMS MATTER

"We delight in the beauty of the butterfly, but rarely admit
the changes it has gone through to achieve that beauty."
Maya Angelou

"Success is liking yourself, liking what you
do, and liking how you do it."
Maya Angelou

"My mission in life is not to merely survive, but
to thrive; and do so with some passion, some
compassion, some humour, and some style."
Maya Angelou

I warmly wish you all the best in self-compassionately
living your restorative, purposeful and meaningful
life full of energy, enjoyment and flourishing.
May you and your children thrive!
With Love
Jo-Anne Henderson

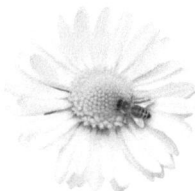

www.ingramcontent.com/pod-product-compliance
Lightning Source LLC
Chambersburg PA
CBHW061138030426
42334CB00004B/85